Spirituality a[...]
in Psychiatric [...]

Stories of Mind and Soul

# Spirituality and Narrative in Psychiatric Practice

Stories of Mind and Soul

Edited by Christopher C. H. Cook,
Andrew Powell and Andrew Sims

RCPsych Publications

© The Royal College of Psychiatrists 2016

RCPsych Publications is an imprint of the Royal College of Psychiatrists,
21 Prescot Street, London E1 8BB
http://www.rcpsych.ac.uk

All rights reserved. No part of this book may be reprinted or reproduced or utilised in any form or by any electronic, mechanical, or other means, now known or hereafter invented, including photocopying and recording, or in any information storage or retrieval system, without permission in writing from the publishers.

British Library Cataloguing-in-Publication Data.
A catalogue record for this book is available from the British Library.
ISBN 978-1-909726-45-1

Distributed in North America by Publishers Storage and Shipping Company.

The views presented in this book do not necessarily reflect those of the Royal College of Psychiatrists, and the publishers are not responsible for any error of omission or fact.

The Royal College of Psychiatrists is a charity registered in England and Wales (228636) and in Scotland (SC038369).

Printed by Bell & Bain Limited, Glasgow, UK.

# Contents

| | | |
|---|---|---|
| List of contributors | | vii |
| Foreword | | ix |
| Preface | | xi |
| 1 | Narrative in psychiatry, theology and spirituality<br>*Christopher C. H. Cook* | 1 |
| 2 | Spirituality and transcultural narratives<br>*Simon Dein* | 14 |
| 3 | Psychopathology and the clinical story<br>*Andrew Sims* | 25 |
| 4 | Helping patients tell their story: narratives of body, mind and soul<br>*Andrew Powell* | 39 |
| 5 | Gods lost and found: spiritual coping in clinical practice<br>*James Lomax and Kenneth I. Pargament* | 53 |
| 6 | Stories of joy and sorrow: spirituality and affective disorder<br>*Frederic C. Craigie, Jr* | 67 |
| 7 | Stories of fear: spirituality and anxiety disorders<br>*Chris Williams* | 82 |
| 8 | Stories of transgression: narrative therapy with offenders<br>*Gwen Adshead* | 94 |
| 9 | Narratives of transformation in psychosis<br>*Isabel Clarke with Katie Mottram, Satyin Taylor and Hilary Pegg* | 108 |
| 10 | My story: a spiritual narrative<br>*Jo Barber* | 121 |
| 11 | God's story revealed in the human story<br>*Beaumont Stevenson* | 132 |
| 12 | Meaning without 'believing': attachment theory, mentalisation and the spiritual dimension of analytical psychotherapy<br>*Jeremy Holmes* | 145 |

| | | |
|---|---|---|
| 13 | Stories of living with loss: spirituality and ageing<br>*John Wattis and Steven Curran* | 160 |
| 14 | Beginnings and endings<br>*Christopher C. H. Cook, Andrew Powell and Andrew Sims* | 173 |
| Index | | 185 |

# List of contributors

**Gwen Adshead**   Forensic psychiatrist and psychotherapist. She trained at St George's Hospital and at the Institute of Psychiatry, King's College London. She is a qualified group analyst and also trained in mindfulness-based cognitive therapy

**Jo Barber**   Mental health service user and researcher with Birmingham and Solihull NHS Mental Health Foundation Trust. She is a medical doctor, although not now in clinical practice

**Isabel Clarke**   Consultant Clinical Psychologist, Southern Health NHS Foundation Trust

**Christopher C. H. Cook**   Professor of Spirituality, Theology & Health at Durham University, Honorary Minor Canon at Durham Cathedral, and Honorary Consultant Psychiatrist in the NHS

**Frederic C. Craigie, Jr**   Psychologist at the Consulting Faculty, Maine-Dartmouth Family Medicine Residency, and Visiting Associate Professor at the Arizona Center for Integrative Medicine, Univeristy of Arizona College of Medicine

**Steven Curran**   Visiting Professor at the School of Human and Health Sciences, University of Huddersfield, and Consultant in Old Age Psychiatry, South West Yorkshire Partnership NHS Foundation Trust, Wakefield

**Simon Dein**   Honorary Professor at Durham University and a Visiting Professor in Social Anthropology at Goldsmiths, Unviersity of London

**Jeremy Holmes**   Psychoanalytic psychotherapist, attachment theorist and Visiting Professor at the Department of Psychology, University of Exeter

**James Lomax**   Associate Chairman, Director of Educational Programs, Karl Menninger Chair of Psychiatric Education, and Brown Foundation Chair, Psychoanalysis, Baylor College of Medicine, Houston, Texas

**Katie Mottram**   A person with lived experience and Inaugural Director of the International Spiritual Emergence Network

**Kenneth I. Pargament**   Clinical Psychologist and Professor Emeritus in the Department of Psychology at Bowling Green State University, Ohio

# CONTRIBUTORS

**Hilary Pegg**  A person with lived experience who contributes to her local NHS trust's spirituality teaching

**Andrew Powell**  Founding Chair, Spirituality and Psychiatry Special Interest Group of the Royal College of Psychiatrists and former consultant psychotherapist and senior lecturer

**Andrew Sims**  Author of the first three editions of *Symptoms in the Mind: An Introduction to Descriptive Psychopathology 1988–2008*

**Canon Beaumont Stevenson**  Group Analyst and Pastoral Care Adviser, Diocese of Oxford

**Satyin Taylor**  A person with lived experience, NHS mental health services chaplain and trainee in the peer-supported Open Dialogue approach

**John Wattis**  Visiting Professor of Old Age Psychiatry, School of Human and Health Sciences, University of Huddersfield, and retired consultant psychiatrist

**Chris Williams**  Professor of Psychosocial Psychiatry, University of Glasgow, and President of the British Association for Behavioural and Cognitive Psychotherapies

# Foreword

I read this book with fascination and interest, and it confirmed my feeling that storytelling is central to psychiatric practice, alongside a deep respect for the patient's own spiritual journey. Two contemporary themes have been employed by the editors to enable psychiatrists better to understand – and therefore be more effective in the treatment of – their patients. First, the spiritual and religious concerns of patients, after years of neglect by psychiatry, have now been accepted as an integral part of psychiatric assessment and care. Second, there has been much recent interest from many quarters, including psychiatry, in the nature and application of narrative – what it is, how it affects the relationship with, and between, our patients, and how it makes for better treatment. These dual themes are maintained throughout this book, which is written for mental health professionals, hospital chaplains and others interested in the relationship of mental health to spirituality. The practical rather than theoretical is underscored, emphasising how users, carers and relatives can all enlist spirituality and narrative for their well-being.

The fourteen chapters range widely over different areas of psychiatric practice and theoretical viewpoint. Most are written by psychiatrists whose primary role has been the care of patients. Transcultural psychiatry is shown to be intimately involved with both narrative and the person's spiritual and religious convictions. Descriptive psychopathology depends entirely on the patient's story, which often includes their spiritual and religious understanding. Psychotherapy is greatly enriched by taking into account the spiritual aspects of life; story is pre-eminent, with narrative an essential aspect of therapy. Other chapters discuss the core psychiatric problems of depression, anxiety, psychosis, psychiatry of old age and mentally ill offenders, in all of which the interweaving themes of narrative and spirituality are prominent. There are moving stories from both a service user and from people seeking help from a mental health chaplain that show the significance of their beliefs in aiding the recovery process. Each of the chapter authors make the case for the significance of spirituality and narrative in their area of mental healthcare and in the concluding chapter, which reviews the book as a whole, the editors summarise the clinical need for taking into account both story and personal spirituality.

I am pleased to commend this book most warmly, and I trust that it will play its part in affirming a spirituality of listening as central to the delivery of good psychiatric practice.

*Baroness Sheila Hollins*
*Past President of the Royal College of Psychiatrists*

# Preface

*Spirituality and Psychiatry* was published by RCPsych Publications in 2009. As editors of that volume, we have been gratified to note its warm reception and that the book was felt to have made a constructive contribution to the debate about the place of spirituality in contemporary clinical practice. So why, 6 years on, might it be timely for a further volume on the topic?

First, we are aware that there were gaps and omissions in *Spirituality and Psychiatry*. For example, it did not have much to say about affective disorders or about forensic psychiatry, and it did not have an author who wrote as an identified user of mental health services.

Second, while *Spirituality and Psychiatry* sought to be relevant to clinical practice and included a series of case histories, we realised in the course of our work as editors that it presented more questions than answers in relation to good practice in this newly developing field. Issues raised by spirituality in mental healthcare continue to be the subject of controversy, and we therefore felt that a second volume, with a different approach, could helpfully further the debate.

Third, while the evidence base has continued to grow steadily over the past 6 years, an important theme to emerge concerns the management of professional and ethical boundaries relating to spirituality and faith in clinical practice. There is therefore a need for a book that is cognisant of recent research literature, but which is also anchored in the realities of clinical practice. The present volume does not seek to review the recent quantitative research literature, although most contributors have made at least some reference to it. It does seek to address the realities of clinical practice in the context of the ongoing professional debate.

Fourth, for service users, spirituality and faith are closely connected with questions of relationship, transcendence and finding meaning and purpose in life – all of these questions being often best explored by way of narrative (or story). Narrative has provided an important theme in recent years in both medicine (Greenhalgh & Hurwitz, 1998; Roberts & Holmes, 1999; Engel et al, 2008) and theology (Loughlin, 1999). Yet to our knowledge, narrative has not been employed as a framework for exploring the importance and challenge of spirituality and religion in clinical psychiatric practice.

This book is intended to ground the abstract concept of spirituality in day-to-day clinical work, drawing on case illustrations to show how spiritual concerns/difficulties impact on, or can be included in, a range of treatment options. We have striven to be alert to the current controversies in this field, while using narrative as a tool for exploring the ethical and professional dilemmas that are raised.

As with *Spirituality and Psychiatry*, the list of authors contributing to this volume reveals a predominance of psychiatrists. We are conscious that we are writing within the profession for colleagues who want to know how other psychiatrists approach these matters, and we explicitly hope to exert a positive influence on psychiatric practice. However, we also have a wider readership in mind, and have invited and received valued contributions from service users, chaplains and clinical psychologists. Some of the contributing psychiatrists have further expert knowledge of anthropology, psychotherapy and theology, enriching the overall account that is provided here – a breadth of input that we hope will additionally appeal to a multi-professional and lay readership.

After opening with an introductory chapter on narrative in psychiatry, theology and spirituality, the chapters explore a range of perspectives on narrative, taking into account the identity of the narrator, the content of the narrative, the therapeutic aim and, not least, the interpretive skills required of the listener (especially the clinician as listener to the narrative of the patient). Chapter 2 considers how culture influences both the narrative related by the narrator and the frame of interpretation required of the listener. Chapter 3 examines how spiritual/religious experience and psychopathology may both be identified within the clinical narrative. Chapter 4 reveals the attentive presence of the clinician as an important, potentially therapeutic aid to the relating of 'narratives of the soul'. In Chapter 5, narrative is presented as a medium within which positive and negative spiritual coping skills can be identified.

In Chapters 6 to 10, different narrative themes are in turn addressed, specifically those of joy and sorrow (in affective disorder), fear and anxiety, transgression and offending (in forensic psychiatry), and experience of psychosis. The different perspectives presented here – by clinicians and patients, and by those who might not consider themselves to be suffering from any psychiatric illness – reveal that narrative can be an important medium of presentation of psychopathology, a means of therapy, a place of finding meaning and a source of healing.

Chapters 11 and 12 present the contrasting accounts of a mental health chaplain for whom the Divine story is intimately reflected in the human story, and a psychiatrist who, as an 'agnostic atheist', recognises nonetheless how spiritual themes are woven into the fabric of dynamic psychotherapy.

These chapters demonstrate that in the telling of spiritual stories, while religion is important for some people, for others a non-religious perspective is to be preferred.

Chapter 13 is devoted to themes of loss and advancing age, and thus to the narratives of older people. Finally, in Chapter 14 we have sought to draw out some of the themes that emerge from the book, and especially the important parts played by beginnings and endings.

We hope that this book may play a part in furthering the telling of all kinds of stories of mind and soul, and that clinicians will feel similarly encouraged to pay close attention to such stories in the best interests of psychiatric practice.

# References

Engel, J.D., Zarconi, J., Pethtel, L.L., *et al* (2008) *Narrative in Health Care: Healing Patients, Practitioners, Profession, and Community*. Radcliffe.

Greenhalgh, T. & Hurwitz, B. (eds) (1998) *Narrative Based Medicine: Dialogue and Discourse in Clinical Practice*. BMJ Books.

Loughlin, G. (1999) *Telling God's Story: Bible, Church and Narrative Theology*. Cambridge University Press.

Roberts, G. & Holmes, J. (eds) (1999) *Healing Stories: Narrative in Psychiatry and Psychotherapy*. Oxford University Press.

CHAPTER 1

# Narrative in psychiatry, theology and spirituality

Christopher C. H. Cook

We all have stories to tell: our own stories, stories we have heard, stories of what we have seen, stories of what we imagine or dream. The telling of stories, and listening to them, seems to be a fundamentally human activity. It is not necessarily the case that happy stories are better than sad stories, and any story can be told well, or badly. But some stories are important and, in some way, they need to be told and listened to. Among these are stories of difficult, traumatic and emotional experiences, stories of life and death, stories of illness. Storytelling is thus at the heart of both medicine and pastoral care. The doctor, like the priest, needs to be good at listening to stories.

If stories are important, the word 'narrative' might immediately appear to be an unhelpful synonym. It sounds more technical and, being employed frequently in academic discourse, could easily be seen to distance the everyday telling of stories from serious academic or professional work. Conversely, it might be understood as a technical term which cuts across various professional and academic disciplines, use of which demonstrates that stories are taken seriously by professionals and academics. This ambiguity is perhaps not unhelpful, for it turns out that narratives, stories, can be told and heard in importantly different ways, some of which are creative and can bring healing, and some of which are harmful and destructive.

## Narrative in medicine and psychiatry

Trisha Greenhalgh and Brian Hurwitz (1998) identify a number of important features of a narrative:
1   There is a finite temporal chronology, with a beginning, a series of events and an end.
2   It presupposes the existence of narrator and listener, whose differing viewpoints influence how the story is told and heard (another narrator and another listener might tell and respond to the same story quite differently).

3   There is a concern with characters, with individual people and with how they feel about themselves and others.
4   Information is provided that is more than simply a definable list of facts directly concerned with events. What is included and not included is important.
5   It is absorbing and engaging, and invites interpretation.

Greenhalgh & Hurwitz argue (convincingly, I think) that narrative is important in medicine:

> 'The narrative provides meaning, context and perspective for the patient's predicament. It defines how, why, and in what way he or she is ill. It offers, in short, a possibility of understanding which cannot be arrived at by any other means' (p. 6).

Narratives provide a holistic and patient-centred approach to clinical problems, identify diagnostic and therapeutic possibilities, are educative – of patient and professional – and stimulate research. Narratives invite multiple possible interpretations – by both doctor and patient – and interpretation offers the possibility of finding meaning. Mutual awareness by doctor and patient of the possible meanings of a particular episode of illness is, or should be, an important objective of clinical practice.

However, narrative is more important even than this brief perspective on clinical relevance might suggest. Narrative, as it emerges in our self-reflection and in our dialogues with others, is increasingly understood as central to the way in which we construct our self-identity (Kinsella, 2006). Because of the power of language, and the social power that doctors hold, it is easy for doctors inadvertently to impose a narrative account which may be harmful to a patient's sense of self. Ethical practice therefore requires a willingness to be self-reflective, to acknowledge in humility the limits of one's own account of things, and the courage to challenge narratives of self or illness which are demeaning, harmful or unhelpful. It also requires the skill of allowing and enabling patients to tell their own stories in ways that are helpful and affirming. Further, there is reason to believe that narratives constructed jointly by physicians and patients have the potential to be healing (Egnew, 2005). Conversely, such narratives also have the potential to impede healing.

One woman, reflecting on a period of mental healthcare experienced more than 10 years previously, wrote:

> For eight years (and teenage years at that) my narrative was challenged by the unadorned, unelaborated threat. 'If you don't obey the System, we will section you and that will make the rest of your life a whole lot harder for you.' That located the authority to provide a correct narrative about me and my self-understanding in the minds of others and not of me, with the full weight of the legal and social authority of the whole state in which I live, subsequently extended to the whole of humanity by the words of the staff nurse, as I said.

Arthur Frank (2013: p. 69) has suggested that illness narratives are a particular kind of self-story, related to and overlapping with, but not replacing, other kinds of narrative of the self, such as the spiritual autobiography, stories of becoming a man or a woman, and narratives of surviving trauma. He identifies three types of illness narrative as aids to listening. In doing this, he stresses that there are clearly other types of illness narrative, and that far from being mutually exclusive these three types of illness narrative are told, repeatedly and in turn, in any particular illness suffered by any particular person. They are: the restitution narrative, the chaos narrative and the quest narrative.

The basic plot of the restitution narrative is 'Yesterday I was healthy, today I am sick, but tomorrow I'll be healthy again' (p. 77). According to Frank this is the culturally preferred narrative (presumably, the culturally preferred narrative of the Western world). Behind it lies the power of medicine to heal, and this in turn takes the focus away from the ill person to those professionals who hold the power to bring healing. It thus silences the narrative of the ill person. A further problem is that this is a narrative of modernity. Once an illness is chronic or terminal, when restitution is not achieved, other stories are needed. These other stories might be potentially helpful but effectively unavailable, as in the case of the religious or spiritual narrative that cannot be discussed with the atheist or agnostic health professional (Cook, 2011). Or they might be available and unhelpful, as in the case of the narrative provided by the staff nurse in the account quoted above.

The plot of the chaos narrative is the opposite of the restitution narrative. Life never gets better. Such stories provoke anxiety and are hard to hear. They are also hard to tell. Frank suggests that they are 'anti-narrative', they lose temporal sequence, they go beyond what can be said, they incur relentless repetition. Although it is desirable to move on from such narratives, Frank sees it as deeply unhelpful to try and rush people along or to dismiss such stories. Interestingly, one of the ways in which he sees this happening is by relabelling such narratives with a diagnosis of depression, a label that enables a shift back to a restitution narrative, the story of a treatable condition.

In the quest narrative, however, the illness is a journey, and the person with the illness, the teller of the story, is afforded a voice in a way that they are not in restitution and chaos narratives, the former because the narrator becomes the professional and the latter because they are almost impossible to tell and hard to hear. Drawing on the work of Joseph Campbell, Frank identifies three stages to the journey: departure, initiation and return. Here, illness is a vocation, which confers a responsibility that the story be told. The outcome is not necessarily restitution, but in this it also surpasses the restitution narrative; it has something to say when an illness is chronic or terminal.

In the field of mental health, narrative plays a particular part in promoting recovery (Care Services Improvement Partnership *et al*, 2007). However, as Fallot (1998) has pointed out:

> 'When the very illness around which recovery is sought may function to disturb mood or to cloud cognitive clarity, the process of consistent meaning making is itself at risk' (p. 36).

It is thus all the more important, and yet also all the more difficult, for people with mental health problems to construct the very narratives that might be expected to help in bringing about their own recovery.

Brown & Kandirikirira (2008), in their report on narrative investigation of mental health recovery in Scotland, have identified six internal and six external elements of narratives that helped to promote recovery (Table 1.1).

Narrative, then, has appeared in recent years to be a useful and important tool for research and for clinical work. However, it also has its potential dangers. Angela Woods (2011) identifies seven:

1. There is a question as to whether narratives reflect real life. Are they true? If so, for whom are they true, and in what situation?
2. Narratives can be harmful – especially if they are used for oppression or dissimulation.
3. The category of narrative can be overinflated.
4. Distinctions between different types of narratives can be blurred. A short case study is not the same as an autobiography, for example.
5. Notwithstanding the work of Frank (see above) and others, there is a lack of adequate attention to the different genres of illness narrative.
6. Researchers and clinicians tend not to be good at recognising the importance of cultural and historical context in the interpretation of narrative.
7. Particular narratives, or kinds of narratives, easily become idealised as the normal or proper mode of self-expression, and thus a particular understanding of the self is privileged.

**Table 1.1** Elements of narratives associated with mental health recovery

| Internal elements | External elements |
| --- | --- |
| Belief in self and developing a positive identity | Having friends and family who are supportive, but do not undermine the narrator's self-determination |
| Knowing that recovery is possible | Being told recovery is possible |
| Having meaningful activities in life | Having contributions recognised and valued |
| Developing positive relationships with others and your environment | Having formal support that is responsive and reflective of changing needs |
| Understanding your illness, mental health and general well-being | Living and working in a community where other people could see beyond your illness |
| Actively engaging in strategies to stay well and manage setbacks | Having life choices accepted and validated |

Source: Brown & Kandirikirira, 2008.

In the context of clinical psychiatry, we might also note that an undue focus on narrative can obscure scientific clarity. Diagnosis remains important for the practice of psychiatry and, at least in some cases, might be obscured rather than clarified by preoccupation with narrative. The clinician needs to see the narrative and the diagnosis, not just one or the other.

## Narrative in spirituality and theology

Spirituality and religion are associated with, and perhaps even constituted by, beliefs, practices, attitudes and motivations that reflect core concerns of human beings. Although it must be acknowledged that some people consider themselves to be neither spiritual nor religious, there are increasingly many people who identify as spiritual but not religious, among whom at least some are atheists (Comte-Sponville, 2008). And there do not seem to be many people who self-identify as religious but not spiritual. It is therefore arguable that spirituality is a universal attribute of human beings, although it has also been argued that this is an imposition of particular Western ways of thinking upon the wider world (Hornborg, 2011).

Spirituality is notoriously difficult to define. A definition that has been used in previous Royal College of Psychiatrists' publications (Cook, 2013a; Cook et al, 2009), and which seeks to be inclusive, defines spirituality as:

> 'a distinctive, potentially creative, and universal dimension of human experience arising both within the inner subjective awareness of individuals and within communities, social groups and traditions. It may be experienced as a relationship with that which is intimately "inner" immanent and personal, within the self and others, and/or as relationship with that which is wholly "other", transcendent and beyond the self. It is experienced as being of fundamental or ultimate importance and is thus concerned with matters of meaning and purpose in life, truth, and values' (Cook, 2004: pp. 548–549).

Such a definition at least incorporates the key areas of debate, and has its uses in clinical practice, but it is not succinct. (Fred Craigie offers some succinct definitions in Chapter 6, 'Stories of joy and sorrow: spirituality and affective disorder'.) The operationalising of the concept of spirituality for research has been understood by some to be so problematic as to be best abandoned, in favour of the study of religion (Koenig, 2008), and moves to address spirituality and religion more widely in clinical practice have been controversial among psychiatrists (Cook, 2013b). However, service users indicate that spirituality and religion are important to them, and that they wish to see these matters addressed in treatment (Mental Health Foundation, 2002; McCord et al, 2004). There is also reason to believe that there is a 'religiosity gap' between mental health professionals and their patients, and that there is need to avoid the misunderstandings that arise as a result of this discrepancy of perspective between the often less religious professional and the often more religiously inclined patient (Cook, 2011). To this end, the Royal College of Psychiatrists has published a position statement providing recommendations for psychiatrists on spirituality and religion (Cook, 2013a).

The above definition of spirituality makes no reference to narrative, and narratives are not necessarily concerned with spiritual matters. However, it should be immediately apparent that there are various important points of contact between the worlds of spirituality and narrative. First, both are concerned with processes of interpretation and the finding of meaning and purpose. Second, both are concerned with how people understand themselves in relation to others, and others in relation to themselves. Third, although it is certainly possible to convey spiritual truths without recourse to narrative, it must be remarked that in many cases spirituality is communicated by recourse to narrative. Thus, many of the great spiritual classics are autobiographical, biographical or allegorical narratives. For example, we might take note of St Augustine's *Confessions*, Bunyan's *Pilgrim's Progress*, and the parables of Jesus. However, we should also note Anton Boisen's (1951) pastoral concern with learning to read 'living human documents' or, to paraphrase here, we might say the spiritual narratives of the service users, patients or other people with whom we work. These are not necessarily written narratives, but they are the narratives of people's lives – recounted to us first hand, or observed by us during pastoral or clinical practice.

The definition of spirituality given above also refers to experiences of the immanent and the transcendent. I have related elsewhere how these dual aspects of spirituality are properly inseparable, albeit differently emphasised and expressed within different spiritual traditions (Cook, 2013c). While an argument can be made that transcendence is a central concept in spirituality, in fact many spiritual traditions are expressed in stories, rituals and other practices that relate to the experience of the immanent, observable, 'this worldly' order of things. The transcendent order, while it may be variously conceived and understood, is almost inevitably either an interpretation of narratives of the immanent realm or else is expressed as an allegorical narrative of the immanent realm (e.g. as in *Pilgrim's Progress*), since something that is completely transcendent is by definition beyond human experience. In our human capacity to interpret narratives we find a place within which the immanent and transcendent meet and are mutually expressed.

Stephen Crites (1971) argues that 'the formal quality of experience through time is inherently narrative' (p. 291). This observation on its own has relevance to the practice of psychiatry, for it reminds us that human experiences are by nature narratival in form. Crites goes on to distinguish within the broader category of narrative between mundane stories and sacred stories. Sacred stories are, he says, 'fundamental narrative forms' (p. 295). They are sacred 'not so much because gods are commonly celebrated in them, but because men's sense of self and world is created through them'. These 'stories within stories' are stories 'which inform people's sense of the story of which their own lives are a part, of the moving course of their own action and experience'. Such stories are 'dwelling places', and people 'live in them'. But such stories 'cannot be fully and directly told'. The stories that actually are told Crites calls mundane stories. In order to be told, stories must adopt the conscious everyday language, narrative devices and imagination of a particular world, or *mundus*.

According to Crites, narrative is fundamental to both our conscious and unconscious experiences of the world. It links us with one another and with a sacred or transcendent order. It frames our self-identity and our understanding of the wider order within which we live. Although Crites does not use the word 'spirituality', we might argue that narrative looks very much like spirituality, or at least that it is the medium within which it can be expressed.

All of this becomes particularly interesting when Crites identifies the strategies that we employ whereby our sense of narrative time is broken. One is to engage in abstractions, whereby general principles are formed that are non-narratival and atemporal. The other is to engage in exactly the opposite process, which Crites calls contraction. Here we constrict our attention to focus on the immediate, concrete, present experience. Both are evident in mental health practice – the former in the abstractions of psychiatric terminology and diagnosis, and the latter in the contractions of evidence-based medicine.

We should note that religious traditions often refer to significant narratives – such as those of creation (Van Wolde, 1996), redemption (e.g. the Exodus narrative in Judaism) or resurrection (e.g. the gospel narratives of encounters with the risen Jesus in Christianity). According to Crites, these are mundane stories – not sacred – since the sacred narrative is the story within these stories, rather than the scriptural or religious narrative itself. However, the study of them, reflection upon them and interpretation of them has traditionally been an important concern for people of faith and this raises a very significant issue. The study of narratives that are important to other people, whether spiritually or religiously or in other ways, is very different to the study of narratives that are important to me. Thus, the study of religion, or the study of spirituality, both of which are important academic fields, is not the same as theology (which usually implies a committed perspective) or spirituality as a *modus vivendi*. A brief excursus on theology and narrative may therefore be helpful at this point, by way of dispelling some misunderstandings about the nature of theology and facilitating a better understanding of what it means to study the religious/spiritual narratives of one's own tradition.

Johann Metz (1973) has argued that

> 'Theology is above all concerned with direct experiences expressed in narrative language... reasoning is not the original form of theological expression, which is above all that of narrative' (p. 85).

All human experience, but perhaps especially spiritual and religious experience, has a narrative quality. Indeed, if we try to avoid this – by focusing too much on the abstract on the one hand (whether that be theological or philosophical abstraction), or the scientific, objective and empirical evidence base on the other, we miss something very important about the nature of human experience. Abstraction and objectification can be ways of avoiding the personal significance of the narrative – whether it be my own narrative or that of someone else. Psychopathology, for example, may be viewed as a way of labelling symptoms, thus objectifying them and using them as evidence in support of abstract diagnoses, or else it may be a means of gaining understanding and finding meaning (see Chapter 3, 'Psychotherapy and the clinical story').

Theological reflection relies quite significantly on narrative, since it is an engagement both with the narratives of lived experience and the spiritual/religious narratives of tradition. The methods of theological reflection are not dependent on the doctrines and traditions of specific religions, but are capable of accommodating the narratives of different faith traditions. Elaine Graham and her colleagues (Graham *et al*, 2005), writing from the Christian tradition, identify seven methods of theological reflection, most of which employ narrative methods in one way or another. Thus, for example, the notion of the 'living human document', takes up the work of Anton Boisen, already referred to above. Or, in constructive narrative theology, the writing of autobiographical accounts – narratives – of experience is emphasised. In canonical narrative theology the narrative of scripture is emphasised. However, all methods of theological reflection necessarily involve some level of engagement between the personal narrative and the narrative of the tradition (in the form of scripture, but also potentially other narratives too). Only the method referred to by Graham and colleagues as 'theology in action' is explicitly non-narratival, in that it sees theology as something to be 'done' and lived out, rather than merely written or spoken about. But even here, the generation of new narratives is an important outcome of the process. Indeed, it could be said that praxis, theology in action, is inherently narrative-creating.

An interesting case, offered by Graham *et al* as an example of constructive narrative theology, is that of Margery Kempe, a controversial English mystic of the 14th/15th century who appears to have suffered a puerperal psychosis, although there is much debate about the most appropriate diagnosis (Freeman *et al*, 1990; Lawes, 2000). According to her own account, her illness (which she distinguished as different from her later religious experiences) included visual and auditory hallucinations:

> 'And in this time she saw, as she thought, devils opening their mouths all alight with burning flames of fire, as if they would have swallowed her in, sometimes pawing at her, sometimes threatening her, sometimes pulling her and hauling her about both night and day…' (Windeatt, 1994: pp. 41–42).

The narrative of Kempe's life (Graham *et al*, 2005: pp. 55–58) affirms a personal relationship with God despite her early mental illness and the later contrary opinions and narratives offered by those around her. Her advisors, friends and acquaintances seem to have been variously polarised in her support or else in opposition to her. Her own narrative (written down by a priest, as she herself was illiterate) is often lacking in temporal sequence and is at times a little chaotic. However, it is said to be the earliest autobiographical narrative in the English language, and it reveals some striking similarities with contemporary narratives of mental disorder, especially in regard to the associated stigma and humiliation of her condition:

> 'Then this creature – of whom this treatise, through the mercy of Jesus, shall show in part the life – was touched by the hand of our Lord with great bodily sickness, through which she lost her reason for a long time, until our Lord by grace restored her again, as shall be shown more openly later. Her worldly goods, which were plentiful and abundant at that date, were a little while afterwards quite barren and bare. Then was pomp and pride cast down and laid aside. Those who before had respected her, afterwards most sharply rebuked her; her kin and those who had been friends were now her greatest enemies' (pp. 33–34).

Margery Kempe's narrative is an account of the meaning and purpose that she finds despite these humiliating experiences. It transforms an account of madness into one of mystical experience (Torn, 2008).

## Spiritual narratives in psychiatry

Roger Fallot (1998) points to seven key religious and spiritual themes identifiable in narratives of recovery from mental illness, which are intended to be illustrative, rather than exhaustive:

1. Whole-person recovery takes whole-person involvement
2. True recovery is a long-term and often effortful journey
3. Hope is an essential ingredient for continuing recovery
4. Recovery depends on the experience of loving relationships
5. The 'serenity prayer' expresses a key process in recovery
6. Recovery is a journey towards genuineness and authenticity
7. Recovery is a story of action and pragmatism as well as conviction.

Fallot understands recovery narratives as drawing primarily on elements of Frank's quest narratives, these narratives involving as they do a developing sense of meaning and purpose that move beyond the limitations of illness and of social stigma. Fallot's work is based on clinical experience with a predominantly Christian African–American population with severe mental illness living in the inner city of Washington, DC. They are therefore not necessarily representative for all other people in recovery. However, the similarities with elements of narrative identified in Table 1.1, based on people in recovery in Scotland, are striking and this raises the question as to whether these are peculiarly religious and spiritual themes, or whether the language of spirituality and religion is at all necessary to convey the key elements of recovery narratives.

Doubtless it is pointless to argue whether or not words such as hope and love are necessarily spiritual. The importance of compassion in healthcare, for example, can be argued effectively without the need to resort to religious language, or even to the language of secular spirituality (Ballatt & Campling, 2011). However, in at least some cases, it is clear that the explicitly religious or spiritual context of recovery does demand a spiritual and/or religious vocabulary. Such contexts are often, but not exclusively, encountered in rehabilitation, mutual help and treatment for people recovering from substance misuse. Many such programmes are either explicitly religious or else adopt the 'spiritual but not religious' approach associated with Alcoholics Anonymous and its sister organisations (Cook, 2010). A recent publication (Sremac, 2014) providing a narrative theological analysis of stories of four addicts who underwent a religious conversion experience during recovery suggested that the traditional Christian virtues of faith, hope and love may be related respectively to the past, future and present realities of these recovery narratives.

In other cases, it is not so much the context that demands religious or spiritual language, as the religious content of the narrative itself, as determined by the narrator. Glòria Durà-Vilà and her colleagues (2013) showed that contemplative nuns who had suffered the trauma of sexual abuse by priests found that the trauma was transformed into a symbolic religious narrative which in turn shaped their sense of self-identity. In particular, religious themes of forgiveness, sacrifice and salvation were important in the process of finding meaning. In a related study (Durà-Vilà *et al*, 2010), based in the same monastery, symptoms that might otherwise have been taken as the basis for a diagnosis of depression were understood by the sisters as being an experience of the 'dark night of the soul'. This study is of particular interest here as it shows how the personal narratives provided by the sisters are shaped in turn by key religious narratives – notably those of scripture and of the *Dark Night* (a 16th-century poem and spiritual treatise written by the Spanish mystic St John of the Cross). An excerpt from one of the interviews illustrates this with reference both to the New Testament narratives of the suffering of Jesus (e.g. Mark 14: 26–42; 15: 34), and to the *Dark Night* (Kavanaugh & Rodriguez, 1991: pp. 353–457):

> 'When I was in my Mount of Olives and I felt abandoned and in despair, crying, I implored God with all my might to take the cup from me if it was possible, this was my Dark Night, my cross and I also cried to God: Why have you forsaken me?' (Durà-Vilà *et al*, 2010: p. 563)

The majority of patients in mental health services are neither engaged in explicitly religious/spiritual programmes of recovery nor as deeply personally influenced by spiritual/religious texts and language as were the sisters who were the subject of this study. Nor, for that matter, are they likely to be living in a monastery! However, either explicitly or implicitly, spiritual and religious themes find their way into the narratives of people who use mental health services and are easily overlooked. It is also the case that users of mental health services have found themselves unable to discuss spiritual and religious matters when they would like to have been able to do so, having feared that such topics will be interpreted in purely pathological terms (Cook, 2011). It is therefore important for the clinician to be able to make sensitive and appropriate enquiry about such matters without either imposing their own personal agenda (or that of a broader social narrative) or avoiding the patient's agenda (Vankatwyk, 2008; Leach et al, 2009; Cook, 2013a).

The woman quoted at the start of this chapter (p. 2), whose narrative had been so unhelpfully and coercively formed by the threat of the Mental Health Act and all that that implied, wrote of how she longed for her narrative to be shaped by what she referred to as 'God's narrative':

> Yes, for the whole of that time I tried to retain a sense that ultimately it's God's narrative that matters, but if we turn to today, a) I don't expect God to have anything at all nice to say about me when it comes to passing judgement; b) eventually I did give up, and I just have very ordinary eating problems (as well as some other problems), but c) the most debilitating thing of all is to get myself into a situation that reawakens the sense of any identity other than the one I strive and fail and long to find in church and before God.

We might debate whether and how it is possible to know exactly what 'God's narrative' is. We might also be tempted to impose a 'restitution narrative' of the form that Frank describes, by way of imposing a diagnosis of depression or of an eating disorder. But I think that the clinically helpful task here is actually to affirm the longing for the self-identity that is sought and owned, and to listen carefully, ensuring that space is given for the story to be told.

## Reflections

Spiritual narratives may convey a theistic or atheistic world view, and they may eschew the language of traditional religion, but they will be narratives of personal experiences, reflected upon in the light of what is held to be most important. The methodology of theological reflection, with the important place that it gives to narrative, provides a way of drawing together such reflections from any or all traditions and belief systems.

It is important to note that narratives can be harmful as well as helpful. A good psychiatrist needs to be alert to ways of helping to affirm patients in telling their own story, and also alert to the narrative (or counter-narrative) that could impede healing or even cause harm. Undue abstraction on the one hand, and excessive preoccupation with the 'evidence base' on the other, can get in the way of the process of listening well to spiritual narratives, which are always deserving of our undivided time and attention.

My first ever publication in a medical journal was a narrative – a story – of my first wife's illness and death (Cook, 1985). Although I did not realise it at the time, I think that this narrative significantly formed my approach to my work as a doctor and perhaps indirectly, after a long delay in time, it also formed my vocation as a priest. It caused me to reflect on illness in the light of what I believed to be most important, and to see my patients, their families and their illnesses differently as a result. It helped me to realise that the real story of illness is concerned with relationships, meaning and purpose, with the spirituality that inheres in experiences of encounter with suffering, death and grief. Of course, there are many such stories, and I have learned also not to expect other people's stories always to be the same as mine. However, when told with honesty, I think that they all share integrity and a quality – I would say 'spirituality' – that binds them together. Perhaps this does not need to be called 'spirituality' – and I respect those who wish to tell their stories under another name. Perhaps they are simply stories of what it is to be reflectively human.

# References

Ballatt, J. & Campling, P. (2011) *Intelligent Kindness: Reforming the Culture of Healthcare*. RCPsych Publications.
Boisen, A.T. (1951) The period of beginnings. *Journal of Pastoral Care*, **5**, 13–6.
Brown, W. & Kandirikirira, N. (2008) *Recovering Mental Health in Scotland*. Scottish Recovery Network.
Care Services Improvement Partnership, Royal College of Psychiatrists, Social Care Institute for Excellence (2007) *A Common Purpose: Recovery in Future Mental Health Services*. SCIE.
Comte-Sponville, A. (2008) *The Book of Atheist Spirituality*. Bantam.
Cook, C.C.H. (1985) Leukaemia in the family. *BMJ*, **291**, 1810–1.
Cook, C.C.H. (2004) Addiction and spirituality. *Addiction*, **99**, 539–51.
Cook, C.C.H. (2010) Spiritual and religious issues in treatment. In *The Treatment of Drinking Problems*, 5th edn (eds E.J. Marshall, K. Humphreys, D.M. Ball): pp. 227–35. Cambridge University Press.
Cook, C.C.H. (2011) The faith of the psychiatrist. *Mental Health Religion and Culture*, **14**, 9–17.
Cook, C.C.H. (2013a) *Recommendations for Psychiatrists on Spirituality and Religion* (Position Statement PS03/2013). Royal College of Psychiatrists.
Cook, C.C.H. (2013b) Controversies on the place of spirituality and religion in psychiatric practice. In *Spirituality, Theology and Mental Health* (ed. C.C.H. Cook): pp. 1–19. SCM Press.
Cook, C.C.H. (2013c) Transcendence immanence and mental health. In *Spirituality, Theology and Mental Health* (ed. C.C.H. Cook): pp. 141–59. SCM Press.
Cook, C.C.H., Powell, A. & Sims, A. (eds) (2009) *Spirituality and Psychiatry*. RCPsych Publications.
Crites, S. (1971) The narrative quality of experience. *Journal of the American Academy of Religion*, **39**, 291–311.
Durà-Vilà, G., Dein, S., Littlewood, R., et al (2010) The dark night of the soul: causes and resolution of emotional distress among contemplative nuns. *Transcultural Psychiatry*, **47**, 548–70.

Durà-Vilà, G., Littlewood, R. & Leavey, G. (2013) Integration of sexual trauma in a religious narrative: transformation resolution and growth among contemplative nuns. *Transcultural Psychiatry*, **50**, 21–46.

Egnew, T.R. (2005) The meaning of healing: transcending suffering. *Annals of Family Medicine*, **3**, 255–62.

Fallot, R.D. (1998) Spiritual and religious dimensions of mental illness recovery narratives. *New Directions for Mental Health Services*, **80**, 35–44.

Frank, A.W. (2013) *The Wounded Storyteller*. University of Chicago Press.

Freeman, P.R., Bogarad, C.R. & Sholomskas, D.E. (1990) Margery Kempe a new theory: the inadequacy of hysteria and postpartum psychosis as diagnostic categories. *History of Psychiatry*, **1**, 169–90.

Graham, E., Walton, H. & Ward, F. (2005) *Theological Reflection: Methods*. SCM Press.

Greenhalgh, T. & Hurwitz, B. (1998) Why study narrative? In *Narrative Based Medicine: Dialgoue and Discourse in Clinical Practice*: pp. 3–16. BMA.

Hornborg, A.-C. (2011) Are we all spiritual? A comparative perspective on the appropriation of a new concept of spirituality. *Journal for the Study of Spirituality*, **1**, 249–68.

Kavanaugh, K. & Rodriguez, O. (1991) *The Collected Works of St John of the Cross*. Institute of Carmelite Studies.

Kinsella, E.A. (2006) Constructions of self: ethical overtones in surprising locations. In *The Self in Health and Illness: Patients, Professionals and Narrative Identity* (eds F. Rapport & P. Wainwright): pp. 21–31. Radcliffe.

Koenig, H.G. (2008) Concerns about measuring 'spirituality' in research. *Journal of Nervous and Mental Disease*, **196**, 349–55.

Lawes, R. (2000) Psychological disorder and the autobiographical impulse in Julian of Norwich, Margery Kempe and Thomas Hoccleve. In *Writing Religious Women: Female Spiritual and Textual Practices in Late Medieval England* (eds D. Renevey & C. Whitehead): pp. 217–43. University of Wales Press.

Leach, M.M., Aten, J.D., Wade, N.G., *et al* (2009) Noting the importance of spirituality during the clinical intake. In *Spirituality and the Therapeutic Process: A Comprehensive Resource from Intake to Termination* (eds J.D. Aten & M.M. Leach): pp. 75–91. American Psychological Association.

McCord, G., Gilchrist, V.J., Grossman, S.D., *et al* (2004) Discussing spirituality with patients: a rational and ethical approach. *Annals of Family Medicine*, **2**, 356–61.

Mental Health Foundation (2002) *Taken Seriously: The Somerset Spirituality Project*. Mental Health Foundation.

Metz, J.B. (1973) A short apology of narrative. *Concilium*, **9**, 84–96.

Sremac, S. (2014) Faith, hope, and love. *Practical Theology*, **7**, 34–49.

Torn, A. (2008) Margery Kempe: madwoman or mystic – a narrative approach to the representation of madness and mysticism in medieval England. In *Narrative and Fiction: An Interdisciplinary Approach* (ed. A. Torn): pp. 79–89. University of Huddersfield.

Van Wolde, E. (1996) *Stories of the Beginning: Genesis 1–11 and Other Creation Stories*. SCM Press.

Vankatwyk, P.L. (2008) God-talk in therapeutic conversation. *Journal of Pastoral Care and Counseling*, **62**, 63–70.

Windeatt, B.A. (ed.) (1994) *The Book of Margery Kempe*. Penguin.

Woods, A. (2011) The limits of narrative: provocations for the medical humanities. *Medical Humanities*, **37**, 73–8.

CHAPTER 2

# Spirituality and transcultural narratives

Simon Dein

> 'Once the patient's biography becomes part of the care, the possibility that therapy will dehumanise the patient, stripping him of what is unique to his illness experience becomes much less likely' (Kleinman, 1988: p. 237).

In this chapter I shall examine transcultural (including religious) narratives of mental illness. I will illustrate my arguments through a number of narrative case studies deriving from my work as a cultural psychiatrist in London (the cases have been modified to maintain anonymity). I shall discuss the clinical implications of eliciting cultural narratives and the ways in which culturally sensitive clinicians can reconcile cultural/spiritual and biomedical narratives and the role of religious professionals in this process.

## Cross-cultural narratives of mental illness

While anthropologists continue to argue over the meaning of the term 'culture', it broadly refers to the shared beliefs and social practices of a specific group of people. Larkey & Hecht (2010) note that the content and delivery of narratives (including conversation, stories, written words, etc.) enact identities and weave together a set of beliefs, norms and values that reflect the culture within which they reside. Stories always have a 'cultural locus' (Denzin, 1989: p. 73), without reference to which they cannot be understood. They incorporate themes, symbols, metaphors and causal attributions which can be understood in a culturally specific way, and which shape the lived experience of illness through the embodiment of cultural meanings.

There are anthropological studies that explore narratives of mental illness in non-Western cultures illustrating the ways in which symbols, metaphors and experiences typically 'run together' for the members of a society. One such example is by Good (1977), who examined 'heart distress' in Iran. People who had experienced adverse life events typically reported sensations of their heart pounding, quivering or feeling 'pressed'. The emphasis on the heart derives from Galenic/Islamic medicine, which is popular in Iran and considers the heart an organ of affect rather than as a means of circulation of blood. These sensations are often closely tied to affective symptoms, including anxiety and sadness, and feelings of being trapped.

Culture-specific stressors include the problems associated with female sexuality, the subordinate status of women, menstruation and bleeding, experiences of family conflicts and loss. Women, for instance, complain that the contraceptive pill can cause heart distress. Thus these somatic symptoms, which they commonly incorporated into their narratives, held specific meaning for Iranians and the authors suggests a close relation between heart distress and Western depression. Good (1977) presents the story of Mrs B.

> 'In the spring of 1974 Mrs B's husband's mother suffered a stroke, was eventually moved to Tehran Hospital and died there. After her mother-in-law's death she complained of depression, a sensation of her heart being squeezed, weak nerves and colitis pains. These symptoms were exacerbated by the fact that her husband had been smoking opium. She consulted several "nerve doctors" who prescribed tranquillisers to no avail. She narrated:
>
> "Finally when I went to the last one, he asked what was wrong with me. I began to cry and told him about my fears for my husband, about my anger and about my youth. When I was a student I was both teaching and going to the university. My father died during this time, but I was able to continue to work and to go to the university. As I talked about my anger towards my husband I began to feel better"' (p. 35).

The expression of emotional distress through heart symptoms is commonplace in the narratives of other non-Western groups such as South Asians. Krause (1989) discusses 'sinking heart' among Punjabis living in Bedford, UK. 'Sinking heart' is an illness in which physical sensations in the heart or in the chest are experienced, thought to be caused by excessive heat, exhaustion, worry and/or social failure. It is based on culturally specific ideas about the person, the self and the heart, and on the assumption that physical, emotional and social symptoms of pathology accompany each other.

## Spiritual and religious narratives

In non-Western cultures, narratives of emotional distress often focus on religious and spiritual themes that place suffering in a transcendent context, providing accounts of the 'why' rather than the 'how' of this suffering, and ways of dealing with it. Emotional distress becomes reframed as a religious narrative which may differ significantly from biomedical narratives. As Cinnirella & Loewenthal (1999: p. 505) note: 'There is growing evidence of a large body of religiously-based beliefs and practices in different groups, which may complement or conflict with those of Orthodox medicine and psychiatry' (see Bhugra, 1992; el Azayem & Hedayat-Diba 1994; Littlewood & Dein, 1995).

Whereas Westerners tend to attribute illness to natural/individual causes, non-Westerners are more likely to attribute illness to supernatural or social causes (Furnham & Baguma, 1999). For example, in relation to mental illness West Africans expect health practitioners to provide spiritual explanations for their distress (Madge, 1998). Chipfakacha (1994) notes that many black South Africans attribute illness to 'superstitious' causes, including spirit possession and magic. Religion and spirituality provide overarching frameworks for drawing meaning that can facilitate coping with emotional distress (although in some cases exacerbating distress) (Exline, 2013). However, it is important to point out that in many instances religious/spiritual and biomedical/scientific narratives are expressed simultaneously and are not necessarily mutually exclusive.

Culture and religion are inextricably woven together (Geertz, 1973; Loewenthal, 2009). Furthermore, the concepts of religion, spirituality, coping, belief and mental illness are themselves culturally constructed (Dein *et al*, 2012; Dein 2013*a*). In this vein, anthropologists have argued that religion is a specific Western term referring to Protestant Christianity and that its cross-cultural use is problematic (Ruel, 1982).

Spirituality, often understood in Western cultures as the sense of connectedness with the Divine, may be conceptualised differently elsewhere. For instance, spirituality in Islam has another meaning. To understand this, one needs to know that there are two separate entities that characterise each individual. These are the *ruh* (the soul), which is the pure spirit (through God) and the *nafs*, attached or intertwined with the living human being, comprising the mortal human's desires, also referred to as the 'lower self'. Attaining spirituality in Islam involves the *ruh* seeking to attain a higher level and attain closeness to Allah (God) through piety and abstinence of negative influences or base desires. This means rejecting the base desires and remaining abstinent from the attraction of the ephemeral world. The *nafs* is the invisible force which pushes man towards good or evil depending on the stage achieved by the individual (Khan, 2009).

While much literature suggests that religiosity, on balance, improves mental health (Koenig *et al*, 2012), cultural factors add a further level of complexity. We should not assume that cultures are homogeneous. Within all cultural groups there are subcultures whose beliefs systems differ from the majority and it is important to avoid cultural stereotyping in assuming that all individuals within a cultural group maintain the same beliefs and practices.

## Narratives in clinical practice

Kleinman (1988) is critical of clinicians for focusing on disease rather than documenting the experience of illness, and in relation to chronic illness argues for 'a sensitive solicitation of the patients' and families' stories of illness, the assembling of a mini-ethnography of the changing context of chronicity' (p. 10) as 'a core task in the work of doctoring' (p. xiii). Moving beyond the conventional history-taking approach in mainstream psychiatry and its emphasis on 'diagnosis', much of my work involves eliciting the stories of those who consult me, to understand the meanings that clients derive from their cultural and religious backgrounds. Pargament (2007) points out that it can be difficult for clients to discuss spirituality; everyday language seems inadequate to the task. However, spirituality can be communicated through narrative; these stories contain symbols, metaphors and images which point beyond themselves to deeper meanings. It is through eliciting these meanings that I am able to work therapeutically with patients.

As Benson and colleagues (2010) point out, 'for refugees, who not only have cross-cultural hurdles to overcome but who also struggle with a higher burden of mental health issues, narrative can offer a method for addressing existential qualities such as inner hurt, despair, hope, grief, and moral pain which frequently accompany, and may even constitute, people's illnesses' (p. 3). I begin with narratives of mental illness among East London Bangladeshis.

## Bangladeshi narratives of mental illness

The UK Bangladeshi population mainly derives from rural Sylhet. They are one of the poorest ethnic minority groups in the UK, with high indices of social and economic deprivation. The majority are Sunni Muslims. Many maintain beliefs in the power of malevolent supernatural forces in the causation of mental illness (witchcraft, jinn[1] possession and 'evil eye'). To seek help, they frequently consult local traditional healers who utilise Qur'anic recitations (*ruquya*) and the ingestion of holy water, although it appears that younger members of the community are increasingly expressing ambivalence towards these ideas (Dein *et al*, 2008). For members of this community, prayer and reading Qur'anic verses are held to strengthen them and provide protection against further attack. Narratives pertaining to what Western psychiatrists would call mental illness typically contain religious and spiritual themes, as in this example:

> Ayesha is a 37-year-old woman from Sylhet in Bangladesh. She came to the UK at the age of 18 and married her husband Mohammed shortly after. The couple have three children, aged 3 years, 2 years and 6 months. The family live in an overcrowded flat in East London.
>
> For several months Ayesha had become increasingly withdrawn, spending a lot of time in bed and refusing to eat. She had lost 2 stone in weight. Her family became increasingly concerned about her. Mohammed and his parents were convinced that Ayesha was possessed by a jinn spirit. In an effort to heal her

---

1. *Jinn* is a spirit created by God out of fire. Jinns have free will and may be mischievous, evil or benign.

they consulted a local mullah who 'diagnosed' that she was indeed suffering from spirit possession and charged them to perform an exorcism in which he recited verses from the Holy Qur'an. However, this was unsuccessful and distraught they took her to see a famous healer in Bangladesh. After a short consultation he told the couple that Ayesha was a victim of jahu (witchcraft) perpetrated by a first cousin who was envious of their marriage. He told her to drink holy water and gave her a taweez (amulet) to protect her against further witchcraft. This had little effect on her mental state.

After returning to the UK Ayesha continued to deteriorate. She was hardly eating and drinking and spent most of the day in her bed neglecting the family. Following a visit from the local community mental health team (CMHT) she was admitted formally to her local psychiatric unit where she was diagnosed with a severe depressive disorder. This was thought to have been precipitated by the birth of her third child and the stresses of living in overcrowded accommodation. She slowly responded to antidepressants and made an uneventful recovery.

In this instance the narrative of distress emphasised spiritual themes, namely spirit possession and witchcraft. While Ayesha remained in hospital, the family were introduced to a biomedical narrative focusing on the role of hormones and stress in the causation of illness. Ayesha and her husband were able to accept this as one possible narrative of her suffering. The art of working with different cultural/ethnic groups is to negotiate between different narratives of illness, in this instance the biomedical and spiritual, and to reconcile them. A local imam with experience of working in local mental health settings attended several ward rounds with Ayesha; his attendance facilitated this reconciliation process. While in hospital Ayesha was encouraged to pray and read the Qur'an to address the spiritual side of suffering. For her, the biomedical narrative provided the 'how' of becoming ill, while the spiritual narrative provided the 'why'.

The next narrative illustrates several points.[2] Biman has predominantly physical symptoms, although psychiatrists would generally agree that he is depressed. Somatization – the expression of psychological distress through physical symptomatology – is a frequent presentation of psychological disorders among South Asians in the UK (Hussain & Cochrane, 2004). As is common in many South Asian groups, individuals and families consult doctors and traditional healers concurrently. Appeal to traditional healers is customary, even though those consulting them may have serious doubts about the validity of the explanations that they provide. Possession by jinn spirits and *bhuts* (ghosts) is commonly invoked by traditional healers who resort to *ruqyah* – supplications using the Qur'an and blowing holy water over the patient to heal them. In an effort to feel better people will make use of what is readily available and are not driven by explanatory models.

Biman is a 27-year-old married man with three children living in East London. Born in Sylhet, he emigrated with his father, a factory worker, at the age of 10 and was educated in the UK. He now works as a waiter in a large Bangladeshi

---

2. A modified version of this narrative has appeared in Dein (2013b).

restaurant. He suffers with depression and anxiety following the death of his father. He explained:

'My father was in Bangladesh, and I was here. He was unwell and I worried a lot for him, and then my father died. During this difficult period, my wife also gave birth to a child – my second child. He had a problem, he used to cry a lot – day and night – we took him to doctors, but they couldn't find anything wrong. The problem was that he would start crying at around 7 pm, and would stop at around 10 am. All night he cried, he needed to be carried and rocked; he would become breathless from crying, and we too used to cry as well. We had another child who was 1 year old at the time, and when morning came, we couldn't sleep, as he was awake by then. The baby used to have foam coming out of his mouth – by the time he had fallen asleep in the morning. Neither of us could therefore sleep.

'During that time, my father had also become acutely ill. He was no longer conscious, and I couldn't go to see him, he died. Four months after he became unwell, I booked the flight tickets for me to go with one of my children, and whilst I was on the plane, my father died, and so I couldn't see him. And after I came back [to the UK], I felt dizzy, and fainted. After this for eight months I felt dizzy, and felt breathless a lot. I used to feel that my breathing had stopped; it used to take me great effort to bring my breath back. This was continuous – the dizziness – even when I am sitting down, not being able to breathe, and even seeing flashes in my eyes all the time, like a blurred TV screen. I used to have pins and needles like my body was heating up, and felt really weak; and when I went to the toilet, I used to feel alone, and that everything around me is moving, like I was losing my breath. It was like this for 8–9 months. Now I am more normal, it happens every day, but it's not continuous like before. And sometimes, I still feel that I can't breathe, that everything is moving.'

Despite consulting mental health professionals at his local hospital, his symptoms largely failed to improve and he became disillusioned with the psychiatric and psychological help (cognitive–behavioural therapy) he was receiving. He consulted a number of healers about his illness both in the UK and in Bangladesh:

'Well, Bengalis say that it's about *tabijs*. I've seen so many *miyasabs* – mullahs (he laughs). They say that a *bhut* (ghost) has possessed me, this and that has happened – and all that nonsense! And black magic and stuff. I have consulted so many *hujurs* – mullah kind of guys who are known to have got high qualification of studying Islam'.

# Jewish narratives of mental illness: Hasidic Judaism

Hasidism is an ultra-religious Jewish movement which centres on the value of 'tradition' and the doctrine that spirituality and revelation is in gradual decline in modernity. Originally deriving from Eastern Europe, contemporary Hasidim are characterised by their mystical and superstitious beliefs, stringent adherence to Halachah (Jewish law), and commitment to the study of Torah. Hasidim had always attributed divine guidance to their *rebbe* (spiritual leader) and a capacity to perform *mofsim* (miracles). In the UK the majority of Hasidic Jews live in the Borough of Hackney, London (Dein, 2004).

Hasidim express antagonism towards the use of psychotherapy and many Hasidim assert that psychologists are ungodly. Similarly, there is extreme reluctance to consulting psychiatrists. Those Hasidim who do seek psychological assistance are frequently diagnosed with severe mental disorder. Hasidim usually make use of psychiatric care 'as a last resort'. Mental illness is seen as stigmatising; those affected have significantly diminished chances of marrying. As Wickler (1977) asserts in relation to Orthodox Jews, the fear and shame associated with mental illness in the Torah community can be compared only to that associated with the most severe Halachic transgressions. He adds that it is often less traumatic emotionally for the family to label their relative as a religious transgressor than as mentally ill.

The attitude towards mental illness, its definition and the understanding of its causes have varied from one historical period to another and from one culture to another. The Torah does not view mental illness either as sin alone or as sickness alone; rather, it has a complex and multifaceted conception of mental illness, including situations in which mental illness causes sin, and other situations in which sin causes mental illness (Wickler, 1977). In the latter case, the penalty for sin is severe (Deuteronomy 28: 15: 'However, if you do not obey the LORD your God and do not carefully follow all his commands and decrees I am giving you today, all these curses will come on you and overtake you (New International Version)'). Deuteronomy states: 'The LORD will afflict you with madness, blindness and confusion of mind' (28: 28). Among the curses threatened for faithlessness to the covenant is that 'the sights you see will drive you mad [*meshugga*]' (Deuteronomy 28: 34). The Hasid with depression may refer to the spiritual tests God set Abraham or the 'weeping prophet' Jeremiah. Thus, depression may be seen as a test sent by God. While in the past mental illness was commonly accounted for by possession by a *dybbuk* (spirit), such explanations appear to be exceptionally rare today (Mintz, 1992). Among Hasidim, illness these days, including mental illness, is frequently attributed to failure to perform a religious observance correctly and it is this aspect that I shall now focus on.

> Mordechai is a 40-year-old Hasidic Jew living in North-East London. He is married with seven children. I was asked to assess him on account of his overzealous religious behaviour. Born into a Hasidic family in north London, Mordechai had always led an Orthodox life, emphasising the study of the Torah and Talmud, the performance of *mitzvot* (good deeds), regular synagogue attendance and celebration of the religious festivals. For over a year before my seeing him, he had been spending more and more time in the synagogue each day, neglecting his personal hygiene, sleep and diet. Of particular significance was his repeating the same Bible passage over and over again, sometimes over a hundred times.
>
> Mordechai's family became increasingly concerned about him, particularly the fact that he was neglecting himself. They asked the rabbi to intervene but to no avail. Mordechai adamantly refused to see his behaviour as problematic in any way, arguing instead that he had committed a grave sin by not reading

the passage correctly and therefore was obligated to repeat it until he believed his recitation was correct. His narrative focused on the relationship between religious observance and sin. Mordechai reluctantly agreed to speak to me and I interviewed him in the presence of his rabbi.

THERAPIST: Mordechai, I'm a doctor, your rabbi has asked me to speak to you. He is concerned that you are becoming unwell. He is concerned that you are spending a lot of time in *shul* (synagogue) and not looking after your family.

MORDECHAI: I am well, I do not need a doctor. The study of Torah is central to our lives, this is what I'm made for.

When asked why he repeated the same passage many times he responded:

MORDECHAI: It is sinful to misread a passage. If I do this, Hashem (G-d)[3] will punish me.

While Mordechai's narrative reflected religious themes, I felt from a biomedical perspective that he was suffering from an obsessional disorder which had a significant impact on the quality of his life. This is congruent with the idea that religion and religious themes are common themes for obsessions (Greenberg & Witztum, 2001; Abramowitz *et al*, 2004). Like many individuals in his community, Mordechai was extremely reluctant to speak to a psychologist, fearing that he would not be understood by someone with a secular background. He refused medication, maintaining that his problem was religious. Sadly his behaviour persisted after I had seen him.

## Charismatic Christianity among UK African–Caribbean

Christian narratives of mental illness focus on three themes: sin, demonic possession and physiological causes. Cook (1997) writes:

'Demon possession and mental illness, then, are not simply alternative diagnoses... Furthermore, demon possession is essentially a spiritual problem, but mental illness is a multifactorial affair, in which spiritual, social, psychological and physical factors may all play an aetiological role. The relationship between these concepts is therefore complex' (p. 17).

Much of the work on the Christian understanding of mental illness has focused on Pentecostalism. A recent study of depression among Pentecostal Christians revealed that even though many attributed their illnesses to demonic oppression or spiritual failure (their illness narrative), many endorsed non-religious explanations such as social and financial problems, childhood abuse and biological factors, including heredity and hormonal imbalance (Trice & Bjork, 2006). Consequently, they were amenable to exploring alternative explanations as long as their spiritual beliefs were respected.

---

3. This is a standard way of referring to God by Hasidic Jews.

In relation to African–Caribbean in the UK, there are a number of churches that involve a syncretism of Christian and surviving African practices (Howard, 1987). Loewenthal (2009) notes that the proportion of African–Caribbean in black-led religious groups is said to be high and those belonging are often involved in lively charismatic forms of worship (Cochrane & Howell, 1995). These religious groups provide important sources of solidarity, identity and spirituality with an enthusiastic style of religiosity. This enthusiasm may be misconstrued by outsiders as signs of disturbance. Loewenthal (2009) speculates that such fervent religious enthusiasm may account for the high reported prevalence of schizophrenia among African–Caribbean in the UK.

> I first met Grace while working in London. She was a 30-year-old woman from Jamaica who had migrated to the UK to study business. She had no psychiatric history or drug history. Shortly after coming to the UK, Grace joined a black charismatic Church in north London. Over a period of several months her religious practice intensified to the point that for a couple of weeks she was awake almost day and night reading the Gospels and preaching on the streets. This culminated in an episode where she was involved in a skirmish with a passer-by; the police were called, she was thought to have a mental illness and was taken to hospital under the Mental Health Act (Section 136).
>
> On her arrival in the emergency department, Grace was dishevelled, excited, had pressure of speech and repeatedly stated 'I am a sister of Christ' and 'Jesus is the Lord, come to him!' It was very difficult to distract her from these themes and she was unable to give any relevant history. She was placed on Section 2 of the Mental Health Act and an intramuscular antipsychotic was administered to her, after which she slept for 12 hours.
>
> The following morning, Grace was coherent and cooperative. She recounted that she was in the UK to study and that after her arrival here she had become involved in a local charismatic church. Both she and her pastor maintained that her behaviour had been inappropriate and that she had taken her religious beliefs too far. She reiterated that she was a sister of Christ (meaning a disciple rather than the biological sister). She remained settled on the ward for the next day (without any medication). The following evening she again became excitable and started preaching on the ward. About midnight she went to her room. Tragically, about 2 hours later she jumped from the window and died.

What was Grace's diagnosis? Was it hypomania? Psychosis? Or was she simply overzealous in her religious practices? At such times it can be difficult to disentangle religious states from mental illness and the involvement of a religious professional could have been very helpful in trying to understand what Grace was experiencing.

## Conclusions

The narratives given here illustrate ways that religion and spirituality are central to the narratives of emotional distress in different ethnic/religious groups and how culture affects religious belief and practice. Mental health professionals need to understand these modes of expression and the role that religion and spirituality play in idioms of distress. The challenge for psychiatrists is to reconcile the religious narrative with the biomedical narrative. In support of this, religious professionals may act as culture brokers by working across religious and secular worlds; they are in a position to help mental health professionals understand the normative expression of religion and spirituality for a specific cultural group. Likewise, mental health professionals can help religious professionals learn about narratives of psychopathology. Each group needs to understand the other in terms of modes of expressing distress if our patients are to be understood and treated according to best practice.

# References

Abramowitz, J.S., Deacon, B.J., Woods, C.M., et al (2004) Association between Protestant religiosity and obsessive–compulsive symptoms and cognitions. *Depression and Anxiety*, **20**, 70–6.

Benson, J., Haris, T.A. & Saaid, B. (2010) The meaning and the story: reflecting on a refugee's experiences of mental health services in Australia. *Mental Health and Family Medicine*, **7**, 3–8.

Bhugra, D. (1992) Psychiatry in ancient Indian texts: a review. *History of Psychiatry*, **3**, 167–86.

Chipfakacha, V. (1994) The role of culture in primary health care. *South African Medical Journal*, **84**, 860–2.

Cinnirella, M. & Loewenthal, C. (1999) Religious and ethnic group influences on beliefs about mental illness: a qualitative interview study. *British Journal of Medical Psychology*, **72**, 505–24.

Cochrane, R. & Howell, M. (1995) Drinking patterns of black and white men in the West Midlands. *Social Psychiatry and Psychiatric Epidemiology*, **30**, 139–46.

Cook, C. (1997) Demon possession and mental illness. *Nucleus*, **July**, 13–17.

Dein, S. (2004) *Religion and Healing among the Lubavitch Community in Stamford Hill, North London: A Case Study of Hasidism*. Edwin Mellen Press.

Dein, S. (2013a) Religion and mental health: the contribution of anthropology. *World Psychiatry*, **12**, 34–5.

Dein, S. (2013b) Magic and jinn among Bangladeshis in the United Kingdom suffering from physical and mental health problems: controlling the uncontrollable. *Research in the Social Scientific Study of Religion*, **24**, 193–219.

Dein, S., Alexander, M. & Napier, A.D. (2008) Jinn, psychiatry and contested notions of misfortune among East London Bangladeshis. *Transcultural Psychiatry*, **45**, 31–55.

Dein, S., Cook, C., Koenig, H. (2012) Research in religion, spirituality and mental health: controversies and future directions. *Journal of Nervous and Mental Disease*, **200**, 852–5.

Denzin, N.K. (1989) *Interpretive Biography*. Sage.

el Azayem, G.A. & Hedayat-Diba, Z. (1994) The psychological aspects of Islam: basic principles of Islam and their psychological corollary. *International Journal for the Psychology of Religion*, **4**, 41–50.

Exline, J.J. (2013) Religious and spiritual struggles. In *APA Handbook of Psychology, Religion, and Spirituality* (eds K.I. Pargament, J.J. Exline & J.W. Jones). Vol. 1: Context, theory, and research: pp. 459–75. American Psychological Association.

Furnham, A. & Baguma, P. (1999) Cross-cultural differences in explanations for health and illness: A British and Ugandan comparison. *Mental Health, Religion and Culture*, **2**, 121–34.

Geertz, C. (1973) *The Interpretation of Cultures: Selected Essays*. Basic Books.

Good, B. (1977) The heart of what's the matter. The semantics of illness in Iran. *Culture, Medicine and Psychiatry*, **1**, 25–58.

Greenberg, D. & Witztum, E. (2001) *Sanity and Sanctity: Mental Health Work Among the Ultra-Orthodox in Jerusalem*. Yale University.

Howard, V. (1987) *A report on Afro-Caribbean Christianity in Britain (Community Religions Project Research Paper)*. University of Leeds.

Hussain, F. & Cochrane, R. (2004) Depression in South Asian women living in the UK: A review of the literature with implications for service provision. *Transcultural Psychiatry*, **41**, 253–70.

Khan, A. (2009) Islam and spirituality. Available at http://www.khilafah.com/islam-and-spirituality/ (accessed 2 July 2014).

Kleinman, A. (1988) *The Illness Narratives: Suffering, Healing, and the Human Condition*. Basic Books.

Koenig, H.G., King, D.E., Carlson, V.B. (2012) *Handbook of Religion and Health* (2nd edn). Oxford University Press.

Krause, B. (1989) Sinking heart: a Punjabi communication of distress. *Social Science and Medicine*, **29**, 563–75.

Larkey, L.K. & Hecht, M. (2010) A model of effects of narrative as culture-centric health promotion. *Journal of Health Communication*, **15**, 114–35.

Littlewood, R. & Dein, S. (1995) The effectiveness of words: religion and healing among the Lubavitch of Stamford Hill. *Culture, Medicine and Psychiatry*, **1**, 339–83.

Loewenthal, K. (2009) *Religion, Culture and Mental Health*. Cambridge University Press.

Madge, C. (1998) Therapeutic landscapes of the Jola, The Gambia, West Africa. *Health and Place*, **4**, 293–311.

Mintz, J. (1992) *Hasidic People: A Place in the New World*. Harvard University Press.

Pargament, K. (2007) *Spiritually Integrated Psychotherapy: Understanding and Addressing the Sacred*. Guilford Press.

Ruel, M. (1982) Christians as believers. In *Religious Organization and Religious Experience* (ed. J. Davis): pp. 9–31. Academic Press.

Trice, P.D. & Bjork, J.P. (2006) Pentecostal perspectives on causes and cures of depression. *Professional Psychology: Research and Practice*, **37**, 283–94.

Wickler, M. (1977) The Torah view of mental illness: sin or sickness. *Journal of Jewish Communal Service*, **53**, 339–44.

CHAPTER 3

# Psychopathology and the clinical story

Andrew Sims

A craggy cliff with the rock strata vertical rather than horizontal records some cataclysmic event in the distant past: a story from an observation. So it is also for psychopathology: the method of descriptive psychopathology in psychiatry is informed observation. It links the patient's abnormal meanings and experience to past happenings inside or outside the person – descriptive psychopathology *is* narrative; the clinician is inevitably looking for patterns, and patterns tell stories. John tells his vicar that Satan is blowing a vapour through the village; this gives him a 'screwed up feeling' that makes him attack his family against his will. On careful enquiry of his experience and its meaning for him, a psychiatrist decides that this is a passivity experience and that this young man has a psychotic illness: the story here is the onset of mental illness inside. Another man, Ron, suffers from severely depressed mood and thoughts of suicide. His story is that he was supporting a young family, after his wife left him, on a low income from a small firm making components in the motor industry. The car manufacturer moved its sourcing overseas; the firm went into liquidation; Ron lost his job and his income stopped. He took a loan at exorbitant interest and applied for nearly a hundred jobs without success. After a day working on his house he developed a frozen shoulder and could no longer use his arm. His depressive illness was largely provoked from outside, and with his story this becomes understandable.

## Descriptive phenomenology

Descriptive phenomenology implies informed observation of another's account of their inner experiences and behaviour: what it means to the subject – not what interpretations the observer puts on it; this was comprehensively described by the psychiatrist/philosopher Karl Jaspers (1959). It aims to achieve understanding by looking at the subjective experience, the personal meaning of thought and behaviour of the subject. It uses empathy, feeling oneself into the position of the other, and so understanding involves using our inner capacity, as human beings, for feeling someone else's experience (Sims, 2003); this is contrasted by Jaspers with explaining, which is the process undertaken by a scientist observing an outside occurrence, an apple falling from a tree, and explaining why it falls. Phenomenology is wholly based on the personal story and it concentrates on its meaning for that person. Phenomenology connects the objective assessment of psychological symptoms and behaviour with meaning – the patient's own personal story: meaning belongs to the patient.

Empathy is the essential clinical tool of the descriptive psychopathologist and involves these stages: the interviewer engages in precise, insightful, persistent and knowledgeable questioning; an account is given back to the patient of what the interviewer believes to be the patient's own subjective experience; the patient recognises this as his own experience; if it is not so recognised, then the interviewer continues enquiry until the description is accepted as accurate by the patient.

In psychopathology we look at the distinction between form and content. The patient is only concerned with the content of an experience ('The nurses are stealing my money'), whereas the doctor needs to be concerned with both form and content ('Is the patient's belief that people are stealing from her: (1) factual; (2) a misinterpretation; (3) delusion; or (4) some other abnormal form?'). Content reflects the predominant interests of the patient, for example, a person whose life has centred on money and fears of poverty may believe that they are being robbed. The form indicates the type of abnormality of mental experience, as revealed by psychopathology, and this leads to diagnosis. It does matter whether this belief of the patient is a delusion or not, as if it is, it implies the presence of a serious mental illness.

> A patient at initial interview believed that he was 'at war with the Evil One', that everyone he met was either a friend or a foe, and that devils were discussing him, taunting him and commenting on his thinking.

The phenomenological form categorizes subjective experience and reveals the psychiatric diagnosis; in this case the form was both delusion and auditory hallucination in the third person saying his own thoughts out aloud. The content is dictated by his cultural context, in his case religious. He believes in a continuing conflict with a personal force of evil, and that this battle affects the whole of life; of course, this content would be shared by many Christians, particularly from the type of church he attended. So the form reveals the nature of the illness, while the content arises from the social and cultural background. Only the study of the form can reveal whether psychiatric abnormality, such as delusion, is present or not, and this can only be explored by finding out what is the meaning of the experience for the individual.

What is the clinical story? In what sense am I using the word 'narrative'? In medicine, narrative is sometimes contrasted with evidence: narrative-based medicine (Greenhalgh & Hurwitz, 1998) *v.* evidence-based medicine

(Sackett *et al*, 1997). This is a false dichotomy: the story is evidence and statistical data (which can be manipulated) also tell a story. The practice of psychiatry, especially descriptive psychopathology, is inseparable from narrative: assessment is based on the story (taking a history), treatment requires working through the story (where can intervention be made?) and prognosis depends on resolving the story (if this be possible).

The past can only be 'controlled' by rewriting our story – we all do it and we do it all the time. The present is controlled by determining that it is under our control – this is the implication of an 'internal locus of control' (Myers & Diener, 1996); I am generally able to order the circumstances of my life and this makes me content. The future is controlled by: (a) planning and taking possible variables into account; and (b) having clearly defined aims and goals. In much mental illness there is a lack of personal control. In psychotic illnesses there may be an experience of passivity – parts of life are under direct outside influence. In 'neurotic' disorders there is often a sense of external locus of control – inability to control one's circumstances, the tyranny of inevitability.

## Can spiritual or religious experiences be distinguished from psychiatric symptoms?

Some critics of religious belief have tried to argue that there is no difference – that religious belief *is* mental illness. This has been claimed, with little finesse, by atheists such as Richard Dawkins (2006), but a much more sophisticated dilemma has been pointed out by psychiatrists with philosophical interests: is there really an intrinsic difference between religious experience and the phenomena of psychosis?

Mike Jackson studied 1000 cases of individual spiritual experience from the Alister Hardy Research Centre archive in Oxford, UK; from these, he and Bill Fulford published three detailed case histories, selecting only those which most successfully blurred the boundary between 'spiritual experience' and 'psychotic phenomena', describing these as non-pathological 'psychotic experiences' (Jackson, 1991). When assessing 'psychotic' they used the Present State Examination, a useful epidemiological instrument for quantitative research but not sensitive for an individual case, and certainly not appropriate for a spiritual and non-clinical interview (Wing *et al*, 1974). They debated the relationship between spiritual experience and psychopathology, proposing that psychotic phenomena could occur in the context of spiritual experiences and absence of mental illness (Jackson & Fulford, 1997). They argued that pathological and spiritual psychotic phenomena cannot be distinguished by:

- form and content alone (as in traditional psychopathology)
- their relationship either with other symptoms or with pathological causes (as in psychiatric classification)

- reference to the descriptive criteria of mental illness implied by the 'medical model'.

This was a very useful paper for me as I, among others, was asked to comment, and this has helped to clarify my views (Sims, 1997). When I read the three cases I found no evidence as a psychopathologist that the three people reported were suffering from psychotic illness at the time of the religious experience described.

Jackson and Fulford chose not to use a fourth criterion: the context in which the phenomenon occurs and its effect on the person over time. I shall return to this later. They state that there is 'a need for clinicians to attend to the values and beliefs of individual patients'. That is the essence of descriptive phenomenology in clinical practice and, when applied to their cases, makes the distinction extremely easy.

One of their cases, that of 'Simon', demonstrates the danger of using the Present State Examination in a non-clinical situation. They assessed him as suffering from 'delusion' as he 'knew' that God gave him thoughts and ideas. His, of course, was the experience of many believers from many religious backgrounds in whom no mental illness has ever been suspected. Simon had had a successful life subsequent to his revelation and he had found it to be a life-affirming and beneficial experience.

If one extends specifically religious experience to more generally spiritual experience, the same principles apply. Informed use of descriptive phenomenology does not just record whether the individual uses such an expression as 'hearing a voice' but finds out, through empathy, what that expression means to them. 'Hearing a message from the spirit of the trees' may indicate that the speaker is a poet; without further corroboration it certainly does not indicate psychosis.

Unfortunately, descriptive psychopathology has often been misused as a formulaic method for making a diagnosis – taking the actual words used in the *International Classification of Diseases* (ICD) or the *Diagnostic and Statistical Manual of Mental Disorders* (DSM). Proper use of phenomenology implies ascertaining what this thought, expression, behaviour means to the person himself, irrespective of the words they actually used. Sadly, many people who have described hearing voices have ignorantly been consigned by psychiatrists to a category of mental illness without finding out the personal meaning of their experience or its sociocultural context.

Both mental illness and spiritual experience are frequent in the population and so sometimes they coincide; but it is often possible to separate what arises from mental illness from what is a solely spiritual experience. Reasons for deciding that 'spiritual' experience or behaviour is evidence for mental illness are based on:

- descriptive psychopathology
- cultural and religious knowledge
- the life course of the person
- common sense.

There are several types of behaviour that may be suggestive of mental illness.

1. The person's description of their subjective experience and behaviour conforms with known psychiatric symptoms. From this account, using descriptive psychopathology, it can be recognized as a symptom of psychiatric illness; for instance, it has the form of delusion.

   An in-patient believed with complete certainty that everyone coming to her ward in the hospital nodded in her direction because they knew, in her words, that she was 'a secret emissary of the Holy Spirit'. Her perception was normal; she saw people coming to the ward and, when she looked at them, they nodded in her direction; this happened. <u>Her interpretation of this perception was pathological:</u> immediately she knew what the nodding meant – when people nodded, she knew that they also knew that she was an emissary of the Holy Spirit and were showing her appropriate respect.

2. There are recognizable symptoms of mental illness in areas of life other than religion, for example delusions, hallucinations, disturbance of mood or thought disorder. When a doctor cannot understand the religious conversation of their patient, and wonders whether or not the patient has a mental illness, they could take the dialogue away from religion – which can sometimes be very difficult – and ask about another, more neutral area. On doing this, one psychiatrist heard from a woman with what seemed to be religious delusions that she believed gas was being pumped through her front door and making her sporadically unconscious – this was supporting evidence of mental illness.

3. The lifestyle, behaviour and direction of personal goals of the individual, after this spiritual experience, are consistent with the natural history of a mental disorder rather than with a personally enriching life event: other symptoms are likely to become more obvious. The manner of life, for example, is compatible with mental illness rather than life enhancement.

   An isolated, unhappy young man living on his own without any occupation in a filthy, chaotic, one-room flat rarely left the house; his only friends and contacts were from a nearby church. His religious beliefs were unusual but the way he lived demonstrated psychiatric disorder irrespective of his beliefs; his lifestyle and conversation pointed to schizophrenic illness.

4. With serious mental illness, such as schizophrenia, the statements, experiences and actions may be concrete, physical and not abstract or spiritual; beliefs may be acted on literally. In some serious mental illnesses there are abnormal processes of thinking resulting in a literalness of expression and understanding. Abstractions and symbols are interpreted superficially without tact, finesse or any awareness of nuance: the patient is unable to free himself from what the words literally mean, excluding the more abstract ideas that are also conveyed. This is concrete thinking. For example, patients have interpreted literally, that is concretely, the scriptural injunction, 'If your eye…

your hand... offend... cut it off.' Finding concreteness enables the psychopathological distinction to be made between the disturbed thinking of the patient with schizophrenia and the description of internal experience of a person with strong religious beliefs. A person with schizophrenia, when describing 'Christ being in me', was able to state in which organ of his body Christ could be located.

A person without a mental illness but with spiritual conviction shows quite different characteristics:

1. Religious experiences are usually regarded by the believer as being metaphorical or 'spiritual', whereas with psychotic illness such as schizophrenia the experience is concrete, physical. For the religious person, the physical boundaries of self are not invaded. In fact, the paradox the Christian describes when Christ 'lives in him' is that he is a 'freer' person, more independent of external influences than previously, with an internal locus of control (Jackson & Coursey, 1988).
2. Thoughtful reticence is shown in discussing the experience, especially with those expected to be unsympathetic. The believer, describing a religious experience, will consider to whom they talk, the situation in which this conversation takes place (e.g. whether a private conversation or not, and the words and phrases that will be used are chosen carefully to describe the experience, bearing in mind that the other person may be unconvinced.
3. It is described with matter-of-fact conviction and appears 'authentic'. The experience may be mundane and everyday; the person may express a degree of surprise that they have had such an experience.
4. The person understands, allows for and even sympathizes with the incredulity of others; they may have doubts concerning the meaning of the experience for them. Religious beliefs are held alongside the possibility of doubt; in this they are like other abstract concepts and not delusions.
5. Usually the experience implies some demands upon the manner of life. It would be normal for an enriching experience to be followed by increased dedication and service to others. This way of life is thought to be morally right and appropriate. Spiritual and religious experiences provoke sustained, meaningful, goal-directed and often altruistic activity.
6. The experience conforms with the person's recognizable religious traditions and peer group; one can see certain patterns emerging in different religious traditions.

# Religious psychopathology

Having determined that spiritual (religious) experience and psychopathology (symptoms of mental illness) are not the same thing, we turn to the links between spiritual and psychiatric phenomena. Two important considerations are: how people with religious beliefs manifest their psychiatric symptoms when they become mentally ill; and how people with established psychiatric disorder sometimes express their symptoms in religious terms. These overlap to a considerable extent, but it is useful to retain the distinction.

There is a long-known association between mental illness and religious expression. For example, many religious texts make an allusion to madness or portray cases of mental illness, and these have been of interest to present-day psychopathologists. The Jewish Bible, the Christian Old Testament, contains a wonderful array of stories, some of which are concerned with mental abnormality, and applying knowledge of psychopathology can be illuminating. One example is the story of Nebuchadnezzar from the books of Jeremiah, Ezekiel and Daniel. His 'madness' occurred in the latter part of his reign, probably in mid- to old age (Daniel 4: 28–34, The Holy Bible, New International Version). His illness lasted for 7 months, during which time 'he was driven away from people and ate grass like cattle. His body was drenched with the dew of heaven until his hair grew like the feathers of an eagle and his nails like the claws of a bird.'

This, probably psychotic, illness was prophesied a year before by the prophet Daniel, and was sent by God because the king had ascribed the powers of God to himself. Perhaps his claims demonstrated the beginnings of his mental illness. At the end, 'I, Nebuchadnezzar, raised my eyes towards heaven, and my sanity was restored. Then I praised the Most High...'. What diagnosis would we now give to this mental disorder? The illness has sudden onset with no previous episodes, occurs in later life, recovery is also rapid and, as far as we are told, permanent. The most likely diagnosis would be bipolar affective disorder, current episode manic with psychotic symptoms. Other less likely diagnoses are:

- schizoaffective disorder of the type that used to be described as 'late paraphrenia' – but the onset, course and full recovery make this unlikely;
- some sort of organic psychosis, possibly substance induced. However, there is no supporting evidence and the course is too long for delirium or an acute psychosis, and too short for dementia.

The Bible does not purport to be a textbook of psychiatry and never attempts to present symptoms for ease of psychiatric diagnosis!

## 'Religious patients'

There are no such people as 'religious patients' or 'spiritual patients', just those who have had the temerity to admit their beliefs to a psychiatrist. Quite often they had anticipated that their psychiatrist would be unsympathetic to anything spiritual. This was not groundless prejudice on their part but based on experience; fewer psychiatrists, proportionally, have any religious belief or affiliation than either psychiatric patients or the general population, and the attitudes of psychiatrists towards the beliefs of their patients have, in the past, tended to be negative (Neeleman & King, 1993; Commission for Healthcare Audit and Inspection et al, 2005).

The term 'religious patient' is best avoided. It is stigmatising. It categorises, and thus dehumanises, patients. It implies specialism: a religious patient requires a specialist 'religious doctor'. This is clearly nonsense; every psychiatrist should be knowledgeable, mentally flexible and sympathetic enough to take on board the implications of a patient's beliefs without having to either challenge or subscribe to them. Most patients have some spiritual notions and many have learnt to be reticent in presenting these to a psychiatrist. Those patients who might be described as 'religious' also have non-religious ideas, behaviour and aspirations. These require the psychiatrist's careful attention and so such patients should not be treated as 'different' from other patients (Sims, 2009: pp. 161–162).

Karl Jaspers, in considering the links between psychopathology and religion (Jaspers, 1959: p. 731) noticed the types of religious experience observed in different mental illnesses. He was interested in how abnormal traits and mental illness have affected outstanding religious individuals, and how ministers of religion deal with people whose religious behaviour is coloured or affected by illness. He investigated how religion might help sick people as well as the occasional coincidence of religion and madness. Jaspers makes a distinction between religious faith that is beyond understanding (the content of revelation) and that which was contrary to reason (namely the absurd). Psychopathology is not an arid catalogue of mental symptoms, but 'the subject matter of psychiatry is always a human being *in toto*, in the context of his life history' (Scharfetter, 1976).

Several different meanings could be attached to the term religious psychopathology (Sims, 2009: p. 147–150).

1   The most straightforward meaning would be to take psychopathology to imply descriptive psychopathology, in which the content is religious in nature.

  A long-term in-patient believed that 'spirits of the saints' were talking about her and criticising her to each other. They were compelling her to put little rolled up pieces of paper into separate cardboard boxes in a recess on the staircase.

  The phenomenological form categorizes subjective experience and reveals the psychiatric diagnosis; in this case the form was delusion (persecutory and religious), auditory hallucination in the third person, and passivity experience. The last two would be considered to be 'first rank symptoms of schizophrenia' (Schneider, 1957). The content is dictated by her cultural context, in his case, religious. So the form reveals the nature of the illness, while the content arises from her social and cultural background.

2   Religious psychopathology could mean psychopathology and be believed to have been caused by some aspect of religion.

There are many examples in histories of the saints. William James in *The Varieties of Religious Experience* tells the story of St Louis of Gonzaga (James, 1902):

'At the age of 10 "the inspiration came to him to consecrate to the Mother of God his own virginity... without delay he made his vow of perpetual chastity... He never raised his eyes, either when walking in the streets, or when in society. Not only did he avoid all business with females... but he renounced all conversation and every kind of social recreation with them." At the age of 12, he did not like to be alone with his own mother, whether at table or in conversation. At 17, he joined the Jesuit order. "He systematically refused to notice his surroundings. Being ordered one day to bring a book from the rector's seat in the refectory, he had to ask where the rector sat, for in the three months he had eaten bread there, so carefully did he guard his eyes that he had not noticed the place"' (pp. 350–353).

Melchior Hoffman, an Anabaptist in The Netherlands, was imprisoned in Strasbourg:

'When Melchior saw that he was going to prison, he thanked God that the hour had come and threw his hat from his head... threw his shoes away... swore by the living God... that he would take no food and enjoy no drink other than bread and water until the time that he could point out with his hand and outstretched fingers the One who had sent him. And with this he went willingly, cheerfully, and well contented to prison' (Dyck, 1993: p. 97).

Neither of these men was subjected to psychiatric examination, and interpretation is conjectural. Their behaviour was strange and possibly showed mental disturbance. In both, the abnormal behaviour may have followed an overvalued idea, possibly in the context of abnormal personality. Religion describes the content but not the form for both. There are many instances of Christian mystics being extremely unusual. For example, the 14th-century female mystic Julian of Norwich stated: 'our true mother Jesus, who is all love, bares us into joy and endless living. Blessed may he be!' (1393). However, fortunately for many of us, being unusual is not the same as being mentally ill.

3   Religious psychopathology could be used to describe some unusual manifestations of religious experience that someone, either at the time or later, has queried as demonstrating psychiatric disorder.

In a notorious case in the North of England, many years ago, a husband and wife joined a minority religious sect who practised lengthy exorcisms on its members. At one of these, lasting for more than 24 hours, the husband, a butcher by occupation, through fatigue and over-arousal, entered into a trance-like state. He became convinced that his wife was possessed and that it was his duty to eliminate the devil. He was unaware of anything else – neither what other members of the group were saying, nor of his wife, at first pleading and then shrieking in fear. He attacked her with a meat cleaver, trying to remove the devil from her, and killed her. The psychiatric consensus at trial was that this had been a dissociative state provoked by the circumstances of the religious ritual, and that there was no evidence before the assault, at the time or afterwards of any psychotic illness. He insisted that he was not

4  Religious psychopathology could describe the thought and behaviour of someone who has both psychiatric disorder and religious belief, the two not necessarily connected with each other.

> A devout but unsophisticated man had suffered from schizophrenia for many years. Often he heard 'evil' voices telling him to jump out of the window. He told his mother about these and she, also devoutly Roman Catholic, said to him 'When you hear these voices, pray to God.' This he did, until one day he jumped through the glass, carrying the whole window frame with him to his death below. We know nothing of his final state of mind. He suffered from long-term symptoms of mental illness and, independently, he also had faith.

There is a practical dilemma faced by mental health chaplains and others confronted by someone who is undoubtedly mentally ill and also has life-sustaining spirituality. It is helpful to realize that the elements of mental illness and spirituality are intrinsically different even though totally interwoven. By listening carefully to the individuals and trying to understand by using their human capacity for empathy, the helper can often gain access to the spiritual through the extraneous noise of psychopathology.

All of these meanings could legitimately be described as religious psychopathology and can come in various combinations. It is of practical importance that mental health professionals should make the distinction between unusual religion and psychiatric symptoms. There is a dilemma: delusion may be very religious, religious belief may be very odd.

## The phenomenology of faith

Accepting that belief does not automatically indicate psychiatric disorder, how do people experience their belief? What is the believer's subjective experience of faith? How can this be assessed phenomenologically? This is very different for different people at different times (Sims, 2009: pp. 151–153). The gist of phenomenology, however, trying to understand subjective meaning, is clearly applicable to healthy people – to those without psychiatric disorder.

Whole libraries have been dedicated to religious experience. It is not my intention to dispose of this topic in a few lines but to show how phenomenological method is useful in understanding what faith means for, and how it is experienced by, the believer. By analysing the phenomenology of religious experience, we can better understand what this experience means and therefore what action may follow.

Only the cognitive, affective, volitional and behavioural aspects will be considered. Cognition includes thinking and believing; the word belief is cognitive – involving rational thought. The religious cognitions of many believers have often been summarized in creedal statements: 'I believe in God...'. This is fine for establishing uniformity, but in practice each individual will interpret the basic words with their own personal meaning. They will also associate the solely cognitive side with relational, affective and volitional aspects: 'My belief in God gives me a feeling of belonging'; 'Belief in God affects what I do, it gives me a code of behaviour'.

Each of cognitive, affective and volitional aspects has implications for self-experience and relationships. Saying to myself, inside my mind, the phrase 'I believe in God' establishes and then enriches the story of what I know about myself and who I am in terms of awareness of being and existing, of being capable of action, of being one person and always the same person, being able to distinguish what is myself from the outside world and all that is not the self (Jaspers, 1959; Scharfetter, 1981). Belief in God has a bearing on relationships: obviously the relationship with God, but also relationships with all other individuals. People (patients) do not live in a vacuum; one must include the social milieu, in its narrowest and widest senses.

Psychiatrists tend to reduce affect or emotion into a few very simple descriptions: depression, hyperactivity, anxiety, guilt feelings, and so on. The real world is much more complex, both in range and in the combination of different, sometimes conflicting, emotions. For the religious believer there is a massive and very varied affective element associated with the experience of faith. This does not mean that religious belief is 'just emotion' or that believers cannot exercise their minds and examine the evidence. Faith cannot solely be based on feelings, but neither can it exclude them altogether. The affective aspect of faith also has a relational side; belief implies involvement with God and with others.

Religious belief is volitional – an act of will and willing actions. Cognitive acceptance of creedal statements with affective involvement in faith leads to individual actions and a code of behaviour consonant with those beliefs. Morality is necessarily linked to activity and employment of the will.

Volition is never straightforward; conflict within the self is variously described but universally recognised. St Paul put it: 'I do not understand what I do. For what I want to do I do not do, but what I hate I do' (Romans 7: 15, The Holy Bible, New International Version). St Augustine, while agreeing with Paul, stressed the nature of the divided will rather than the divided self. Cook has developed a theological model about volition for alcohol addiction that can be extended more generally in psychiatry (Cook, 2006). In a sense we are all addicts – to something or to several things. The theological model of addiction, which applies to believers and non-believers, implies that the internal conflict is serious; to be freed from addiction, a second-order volition is necessary – to want-to-want not to drink. The addict needs more than his own willpower, but the grace of God is available for all. Spiritual enlightenment comes in realizing and recognizing this: 'We know that the law is spiritual; but I am unspiritual, sold as a slave to sin' (Romans 7: 14–15, The Holy Bible) We have to look outside ourselves for help to be released from what St Paul calls 'slavery'.

## Phenomenology with spirituality

The previous section concerns 'faith', and by implication, religion. How about spiritual experience without religion? The same phenomenological characteristics are useful and relevant: cognition, affect, volition, behaviour, self-experience and relationship. The profile is still there, although sometimes with less distinct definition.

The 'clinical story' becomes meaningful when it is exposed to phenomenological analysis; at the same time, without a narrative to work on, there can be no study of psychopathology. From Jaspers onwards a spiritual or religious aspect has been indispensable for looking at human experience as a whole person. Psychopathology is only helpful if combined with the social and cultural context; that is wherever the story comes in. To do justice to the patient, we must try to understand.

> Lucy, now 60, has reached tranquillity after many years of mental illness. Her family were not religious, and Sunday school for a few years in her teens was her only early experience of faith. She left school at 16, worked in the Civil Service and 'drifted into marriage' at 20. They had no children and parted after 6 years.
>
> When her father died, the whole family suffered. Lucy became anxious and depressed. She stopped working, avoided other people, did not get dressed and neglected herself. She was preoccupied with thoughts that she was unclean; she kept washing herself and her clothes and taking baths, but this was never enough. She sensed her now dead father's presence in her home. She felt 'my home and my marriage and everything that held me together had gone'. In some way, feeling dirty was linked to sex with her husband, feeling guilty that they had had sex before marriage; she was plagued with guilt.
>
> Her first psychiatric admission, aged 29, was for 1 month. After discharge, she felt no better inside. She started going to church but stopped because she thought that people disapproved of her. A few months later she became 'quite buoyant' and 'fixated on a pop group', believing herself to be in love with the lead singer; she spent a lot of money on clothes, and ate voraciously; she wrote prolifically to the pop star each night, and this resulted in her readmission to hospital, this time compulsorily.
>
> In her early 30s she had several further hospital admissions. She became more regular in her church attendance and found that faith helped her – 'it was something new, hopeful, exciting and could wash away the dirt. I could start again.' She believed that God forgave her and she could make a new life, so that she did not have to continue excessive washing. Her mental health improved over several years.
>
> There have been two further episodes of psychotic illness requiring hospital admission, both occurring after ceasing medication. On one occasion she became 'fixated' on a college lecturer. He reported her to the police and she 'ran away to Australia'. She arrived at Sydney in a bad state, was looked after by a Salvation Army chaplain, admitted to a mental hospital and then transferred back to Britain.

In the past few years she has become a valued member of her church. Her faith has 'always been hopeful and positive… there is no doubt that God's hand has been on my life, He has cared for me and protected me'. She remains on medication.

In Lucy's story, 'mental illness' and 'spiritual experience' can be separated. Lucy has had bipolar disorder with several discreet episodes of illness, in some of which she became psychotic. She came to faith in her 30s, after the mental illness had started and her belief and practice have been positive, giving her a 'feeling of rationality'. Unless she tells her story, the relationship between faith and mental illness cannot be ascertained, nor its value in stabilizing her life realized. Without psychopathological appraisal there can be no psychiatry; without hearing the story there can be no psychopathology.

# References

Commission for Healthcare Audit and Inspection, Care Services Improvement Partnership, Mental Health Act Commission, et al (2005) *Count Me In: Results of a National Census of In-Patients in Mental Health Hospitals and Facilities in England and Wales.* Healthcare Commission.

Cook, C.C.H. (2006) *Alcohol, Addiction and Christian Ethics.* Cambridge University Press.

Dawkins, R. (2006) *The God Delusion.* Bantam Press.

Dyck, C.J. (1993) *An Introduction to Mennonite History.* Herald Press.

Greenhalgh, T. & Hurwitz, B. (1998) *Narrative Based Medicine: Dialogue and Discourse in Clinical Practice.* BMJ Books.

Jackson, M.C. (1991) *A Study of the Relationship between Psychotic and Religious Experience* (PhD thesis). University of Oxford.

Jackson, L.E. & Coursey, R.D. (1988) The relationship of God control and internal locus of control to intrinsic religious motivation, coping and purpose in life. *Journal for the Scientific Study of Religion,* **27**, 399–410.

Jackson, M.C. & Fulford, K.W.M. (1997) Spiritual experience and psychopathology. *Philosophy, Psychiatry and Psychology,* **4**, 41–66.

James, W. (1902) *The Varieties of Religious Experience.* Longmans, Green & Co.

Jaspers, K. (1959) *General Psychopathology,* 7th edn (transl. J. Hoenig & M.W. Hamilton, 1963). Manchester University Press.

Julian of Norwich (1393) *Revelations of Divine Love* (ed. M. Glasscoe). Medieval Texts.

Myers, D.G. & Diener, E. (1996) The pursuit of happiness: new research uncovers some anti-intuitive insights into how many people are happy – and why. *Scientific American,* **274**, 54–6.

Neeleman, J. & King, M.B. (1993) Psychiatrists' religious attitudes in relation to their clinical practice: a survey of 231 psychiatrists. *Acta Psychiatrica Scandinavica,* **88**, 420–4.

Sackett, D.L., Richardson, W.S., Rosenberg, W., et al (1997) *Evidence-Based Medicine: How to Practice and Teach EBM.* Churchill Livingstone.

Scharfetter, C. (1976) *General Psychopathology: An Introduction* (transl. H. Marshall, 1980): p. 2. Cambridge University Press.

Scharfetter, C. (1981) Ego-psychopathology: the concept and its empirical evaluation. *Psychological Medicine,* **11**, 273–80.

Schneider, K. (1957) Primary and secondary symptoms in schizophrenia. *Fortschrift für Neurologie und Psychiatrie,* **25**, 487–90. In *Themes and Variations in European Psychiatry: An Anthology* (transl. H. Marshall, eds S. Hirsch & M. Shepherd). John Wright & Sons, 1974.

Sims, A. (1997) Commentary on 'Spiritual experience and psychopathology'. *Philosophy, Psychiatry and Psychology*, **4**, 79–81.

Sims, A. (2003) *Symptoms in the Mind: An Introduction to Descriptive Psychopathology*, 3rd edn. Saunders.

Sims, A. (2009) *Is Faith Delusion?* Continuum.

Wing, J.K., Cooper, J.E. & Sartorius, N. (1974) *Measurement and Classification of Psychiatric Symptoms*. Cambridge University Press.

CHAPTER 4

# Helping patients tell their story: narratives of body, mind and soul

Andrew Powell

> A patient who was a devout Christian was admitted to hospital as an emergency. She tried to explain to the duty psychiatrist the importance of her belief in 'the Holy Ghost', only to hear it reported in the ward round the next day that she had been seeing ghosts.

In this chapter, I aim to show that the narrative set in motion when a patient is seen by a psychiatrist is not only an account of an individual's life experience but also attuned to the expectations of the psychiatrist – more than either of them may be aware. This is especially relevant to soul narrative, which is often invested with profound personal meaning, yet can lead to confusion when not understood, or else is likely to remain unvoiced if a patient senses that their spiritual beliefs and concerns are not given credence. I conclude by illustrating how the soul narrative, when encouraged, can bring real therapeutic benefits.

## The pre-eminence of medical diagnosis

In general medicine, taking a patient's history is followed by hands-on examination of the body, feeling for lumps and bumps, listening to the heart and lungs and testing for abnormalities of the nervous system, followed when needed by a battery of investigations. The unspoken contract between physician and patient enables doctors to divide their attention between relating to their patients as persons and yet examining their bodies with the detachment needed to identify pathology and arrive at an accurate diagnosis (in Greek, *dia* means 'stand apart', *gnosis* means 'discern').

The art of diagnosis has its roots in the ancient civilisations of Egypt, Greece and China. But the physician of our time is heir principally to a scientific method that began during the Renaissance with the study of human anatomy and which has brought extraordinary knowledge of how the body works. A correct diagnosis will generally indicate a disease that has recognisable pathology, a cause (aetiology), a natural history (it may progress or remit) and an outcome (prognosis). At best, getting the diagnosis right leads to a treatment that cures and if not to a cure, then at least to the relief of symptoms; failing that, quality of care management for chronic illness; and when the condition is terminal, for best-practice end-of-life care.

Making the diagnosis requires a relentless kind of questioning impressed on every medical student and never forgotten: Where is the pain? Is it a dull ache or stabbing? Does it radiate? Does anything bring it on, or relieve it? How about exercise, or eating, or lying down? This kind of enquiry rapidly becomes second nature to doctors, like being a journalist on the trail of something suspicious and digging away until the whole picture emerges. The diagnostic narrative is relatively impersonal, focusing on the elucidation of symptoms and their causes. Yet general medicine has long had to take note of the body–mind connection. We know from psychosomatic medicine, psychoneuroimmunology and liaison psychiatry that in-depth enquiry into a patient's personal life, feelings, stresses and habits may be required. Indeed, some 20% of patients in general practice present with underlying emotional disorder (De Waal *et al*, 2004). Common to all these consultations, however, is the straightforward aim of helping the patient back to physical health and well-being. If body and mind can be likened to car and driver, the driver is being questioned in order to help with getting the car back on the road.

Mental health science, too, has its roots in physical medicine. More than a century ago, abnormal states of mind secondary to nutritional diseases, syphilis, porphyria, hormonal disturbances and brain injury encouraged the search for physical causation. A minority of mental disorders are indeed secondary to organic pathology, as with endocrine disorders, neurodegenerative disease, or where there is a brain lesion. More recently, neurodevelopmental deficits are implicated in a number of conditions, including autistic spectrum disorders and possibly schizophrenia. In the field of intellectual disability, genetic counselling and research are proving invaluable. All of these conditions highlight the importance of psychiatry as a branch of medicine and underline the value of the diagnostic narrative.

## Descriptive psychopathology: a two-edged sword?

Yet it behoves us to question the relevance of physical medicine to current psychiatric practice, for general psychiatrists rarely come across organic pathology. Curiously, the broad acceptance of psychiatry as a medical specialty owes most to Emil Kraepelin's historic classification of the functional psychoses into schizophrenia and manic depression (bipolar disorder) at the end of the 19th century. Thereafter, it only remained for psychiatry to demonstrate the biology of mental disorder. Even so, to this day the aetiology of schizophrenia and bipolar disorder remains obscure. Neurochemical hypotheses having proved inconclusive, new hope is now being invested in brain studies in the search for definitive neuropathology.

The pressure is on, for while the combined prevalence of schizophrenia and bipolar disorder in the population remains constant at around 2%, there now appears to be an epidemic of mental illness, since some 25% of women and 12% of men will need treatment for depression in the course of a lifetime (Mental Health Foundation, n.d.). According to the World Health Organization (n.d.) (WHO), mental disorder currently affects one in ten adults, accounting for over 12% of the global burden of disease and over 40% of the total burden of disability in Europe and the Americas.

Most of these disorders have no clear-cut aetiology and no consistent prognosis. The picture is often a complex interplay of constitutional, developmental and environmental factors coupled with situational stress. Yet the diagnostic narrative in psychiatry, whether using the framework of the *International Classification of Diseases* (ICD) or the *Diagnostic and Statistical Manual of Mental Disorders* (DSM), has been to attempt to define mental illness with the same objectivity and rigour as physical disorders. For the most part it has simply led to the categorisation of symptom clusters. Descriptive psychopathology usefully serves as the lingua franca among psychiatrists, but often has little to say about the cause (and outcome) of the presenting problem. Yet DSM and ICD between them encompass and label just about every aspect of the human condition. The questionable introduction in 1980 of the category of 'major depression' in DSM-III was followed by 21 million prescriptions for fluoxetine (Prozac) being dispensed over the next 10 years (Shorter, 2014) and currently the psychopharmaceutical industry makes annual profits of around 87 billion dollars (Williams, 2011), a powerful testament to the widespread appeal of the pharmaceutical narrative of mental disorder (Davies, 2013).

## Life comes with a health warning

The indelicate quip 'life is a sexually transmitted disease for which there is no treatment and which is uniformly fatal', pinpoints the reality of human suffering, something discussed by psychiatrists less than it deserves, possibly because we live in a culture that prefers a pharmaceutical narrative rather than face up to the travails of humanity. How might we account for the soaring prevalence of mental disorder? Is the human race in decline? Is the world of materialism and consumerism eroding the core values that make life feel worthwhile (Powell, 2013)? Or, as Thomas Szasz suggested more than half a century ago (Szasz, 1960), are we looking at the demographic of a societal narrative that now habitually pathologises the human condition?

These are complex matters and hard-pressed clinicians are not much given to questioning the extent that psychiatry mirrors an all-pervasive societal narrative. Nevertheless, most psychiatrists would agree that the continuum of distress extends from the pain of the human condition at the one end to severe (and often treatable) mental illness at the other.

Yet a fundamental problem remains: much of psychiatry has been built on unsubstantiated premises for which no amount of classification can compensate.

## Dynamic psychopathology: another two-edged sword?

All great institutions have to bear the strain of internal dissent. Psychiatry is no exception, for a competing narrative to the biomedical model began more than a century ago with Sigmund Freud. Freud promised a new understanding of the human mind in which doctor and patient would join in the search for meaning that lay encoded in the symptom; the symbolic life of the unconscious would be laid bare and its arcane mysteries revealed. For the first half of the 20th century, the narrative of psychoanalysis, known as 'the talking cure', reigned supreme in the Americas and Europe.

Central to this narrative is the notion that the therapist listens to and interprets the unconscious significance of the patient's story. The understanding that follows relieves the patient of the symptom by revealing the source of emotions that have had to be repressed, denied or otherwise disavowed, as illustrated by the following example.

> Jean came into therapy with a history of recurrent panic attacks. The attacks intensified each time she entered into a serious relationship that might lead to an emotional commitment, yet she very much wanted to settle down and have a family. In therapy Jean suffered a severe panic attack during a session just before the summer break. With the help of the therapist, Jean was able to explore the significance of this panic, which brought back painful memories of childhood when her mother had to be hospitalized for a lengthy period due to a life-threatening illness. Once Jean understood that her panic attacks were a resurgence of her fears of abandonment, the break could be successfully managed without further attacks. Three years after the conclusion of therapy, Jean wrote to let her therapist know she was now married and mother of a baby girl.

Countless people have benefited from such an approach. However, the outcome is not always successful and there has been ethical concern over the imbalance of power that arises. For instance, how can a patient give truly informed consent when the analysis of 'unconscious' material is the prerogative of the therapist? How free is the patient to disagree with the therapist when this can be interpreted as 'resistance'? What about the risk that the patient's narrative is being subtly appropriated by the therapist and re-fashioned according to the therapist's world view? Seeing all of the human condition through the lens of dynamic psychopathology can result in therapy that is more a way of life than a treatment. Freud himself warned against this danger (Freud, 1937).

Good therapists go to great lengths to avoid the abuse of power. Yet when a professional advises someone in need of help and who is less knowledgeable, the risk is always there, whether it be psychotherapy or pharmacotherapy. The more susceptible the patient, the greater the ethical obligation on the professional. Offering no conceptual map risks leaving the patient floundering, yet a favoured theoretical preconception can trammel a vulnerable mind.

If democracy of spirit is to prevail in the course of a psychological therapy, the therapist must take care not to make conjecture sound like fact (since no one can truly know what is in the mind of another) but rather to invite the patient to respond freely and authentically. No matter how appealing and persuasive a theory may be, authenticity holds the key to genuinely therapeutic narrative. This has to be the touchstone if one's patient is going to find, in the telling, a new, creative and enduring meaning to their story.

## Authentic narrative

In an authentic exchange, the narrative is an act of co-creation. Authenticity requires that both people meet on the basis of equality as human beings, each contributing with their own experience. Therapeutic expertise is able to be valued and acknowledged but it is important to recognise that 'therapist' and 'patient' are no more than complementary roles set up to enable the one to give to the other a special kind of assistance.

Across healthcare, the setting is conducive to a parent/child dynamic because of the knowingness of the clinician and the dependency needs of the patient. In some circumstances this is helpful, but there is the danger of precluding a more valid interpersonal exchange – validity founded on acknowledging that we are all travellers on life's journey, facing the same landmarks, losses, hopes and fears. As Carl Rogers remarked, 'what is most personal is most general' (Rogers, 1961: p. 27); without this awareness no person, however clever and knowledgeable, could reach out and help another.

Especially in mental healthcare, when this authority-based dynamic stands in the way of authenticity, the balance needs restoring; then comes the discovery that each person is writing their own life story and that nobody can be the instrument for change except oneself.

The narrative that charts a person's life from birth through to this present moment must sooner or later find reconciliation with the past, for there is no changing the facts of the story, as the 10th-century Persian poet and philosopher Omar Khayyám wryly reflects (Fitzgerald, 1859):

> 'The Moving Finger writes; and, having writ,
> Moves on: nor all thy Piety nor Wit
> Shall lure it back to cancel half a Line,
> Nor all thy Tears wash out a Word of it.'

What a person *can* change, however, is *how* to relate to those events of the past; whether to remain a victim of circumstance or to see adversity as the grit that makes the pearl. The choice lies between repeating the same chapter over and over or starting a new one. Every story must have its past; the life-affirming story has a future too. When the ego, through force of habit, resists change, the clinician can invite a more soulful exchange to lend support, as will be described later.

# The power of narrative for good or ill

A sign of mental health is that a person's chronicle of events and experiences is interwoven to form a coherent and meaningful narrative; 'living' this narrative is an act of involuntary creativity that enriches the self and its circle of intimates. Some people reach a wider audience through the arts, education, business or politics. Not least, the great spiritual exemplars have touched innumerable lives with their uncompromising narratives of wisdom and truth. Of the spiritual teacher, the Zen scholar Daisetz Suzuki writes:

> 'His hands and feet are the brushes and the whole universe is the canvas on which he depicts his life… this picture is called history' (Herrigel, 1953: p. 8).

In contrast, psychotic narrative, while often vociferously proclaiming the 'truth', is likely to be painfully disjointed, or else tragically concrete as in the case of this patient with schizophrenia convicted of homicide, who said:

> 'I took a life because I needed one' (Cox, 1982).

Groups, too, can spawn 'psychotic' narratives in which the individual is swept up by perverse ideology, resulting in horrific genocide as in Rwanda (Ilibagiza, 2006), or mass suicide as in the case of the Jonestown massacre in Guyana (Scheeres, 2011), when Jim Jones, the paranoid cult leader, commanded some 900 followers to take poison to save them from the evils of the world.

On the other hand, surrender of the self to a higher power is a hallmark of religious belief. Speaking in tongues (the 'Toronto blessing') is endorsed by many evangelical Christians as a divine gift. Should such altered states of consciousness be regarded as psychopathological? Not necessarily, according to ICD-10, which under trance and possession disorder (F44.3) specifies:

> '… Include here only trance states that are involuntary or unwanted, occurring outside religious or culturally accepted situations' (World Health Organization, 2016).

In this case, psychiatry must distinguish between mental illness and mental health solely on the context of the event. Here we find a conflation of medical and social narratives that while offering some practical help does little to clarify what is really going on.

What, then, about people who join 'hearing voices' groups, in which many group members will have already been diagnosed as having mental illness? With the help of the group, a new kind of coherent narrative is established, based on sharing the experience of intrusive voices and how to challenge them and find a way to live with them. This may require strategies such as negotiating with the voices and insisting they wait until, say, the evening when they can be promised an hour of undivided attention (Romme & Escher, 1989).

Such narrative has moved away from the concept of psychopathology to becoming a means of adaptation. We might compare this with an amputee who, once the injury has been attended to, no longer regards himself as ill just because he will need a prosthesis.

These various narratives illustrate that 'psychopathology' is context bound and cannot be divorced from circumstance. When a person is deprived under the Mental Health Act of their right to freedom, the narrative is likely to be one of confusion, fear and anger and it may be impossible to engage in meaningful dialogue. The psychiatrist needs to tolerate the anger often shown by the patient, while remaining 'present' to help make sense of the anguish and confusion as it passes. As Professor Larry Davidson from Yale University, USA, says,

> 'Recovery means learning how to live outside the mental illness rather than inside it. To live inside the mental illness is to be lost in its downward spiral. Living outside schizophrenia is about reclaiming your life. It is about self-determination, choice, hope, and empowerment' (Summerville, 2009).

The construction of such a narrative of recovery is a powerful building tool in learning to live 'outside' the illness.

## The spiritual narrative

Psychiatrists face a unique challenge when evaluating experiences phenomenologically indistinguishable from mental illness, yet potentially invested with profound spiritual significance (Lucas, 2011). What distinguishes a person who has an acute and transient psychotic disorder, from one who has what turns out to be a life-changing spiritual revelation? Consider this hallucinatory episode:

> 'Now as [Saul] was going along and approaching Damascus, suddenly a light from heaven flashed around him. He fell to the ground and heard a voice saying to him, "Saul, Saul, why do you persecute me?" He asked, "Who are you, Lord?" The reply came, "I am Jesus, whom you are persecuting" [...] Saul got up from the ground, and though his eyes were open, he could see nothing; so they led him by the hand and brought him into Damascus. For three days he was without sight, and neither ate nor drank.
>
> Now there was a disciple in Damascus named Ananias [...] He laid his hands on Saul and said, "Brother Saul, the Lord Jesus, who appeared to you on your way here, has sent me so that you may regain your sight and be filled with the Holy Spirit." And immediately something like scales fell from his eyes, and his sight was restored' (Acts 9: 4, 5, 8–10, 17, 18, The Holy Bible, New Revised Standard Version).

Would Saul (later renamed Paul the Apostle), had he lived today, been diagnosed with acute and transient psychotic disorder? And what should we make of the risk of recurrence? Whereas many people who experience repeated episodes of acute and transient psychotic disorder never progress to chronic schizophrenia (Farooq, 2012), one in eight does so within 5 years (Queirazza *et al*, 2014). Psychiatry has traditionally looked askance at spiritual and religious preoccupation because of this association with psychosis. Yet the studies of Koenig *et al* (2012) have demonstrated a broadly positive correlation between religion, spiritual practice and improved mental as well as physical health. Given that many people have such 'exceptional human experiences', leading them to a new sense of meaning and purpose in life, perhaps we should not too readily focus on psychopathology for fear that illness may lie ahead.

There continues to be controversy nonetheless. A study by King *et al* (2013) claims to show that religion confers no additional protection against mental disorder when compared with those people who are neither spiritual nor religious. King also unequivocally states that that 'people who profess spiritual beliefs in the absence of a religious framework are more vulnerable to mental disorder'. While King does not go so far as to suggest that 'spirituality' causes mental disorder, it would be easy to draw that erroneous conclusion. There is, however, an important sociological perspective to consider. Contemporary Western society, with its erosion of deeper values and materialistic pursuit of pleasure, avoids asking the difficult questions 'Why are we here?' and 'What it is all for?' If a person is deeply preoccupied with such existential concerns, they may well be labelled as depressed. Yet self-doubt and anguish have always been features of the spiritual life, as instanced by such historic persons as Julian of Norwich and John of the Cross. In the largely secular society of Britain today, there is a burgeoning demographic of 'spiritual but not religious' for whom soul-searching can be a lonely pursuit. Without a climate of understanding or the community support of a faith tradition, the individual seeker may well struggle. Pargament (2011) points out that spiritual struggles have the potential for either good or bad mental health outcomes. So, 'Perhaps the question to ask is whether the world in which we now live is conducive to a good outcome' (Cook & Powell, 2013).

A more radical interpretation has been suggested by Razzaque, who turns King's conclusion upside down by suggesting that the finding is unremarkable, since people who have a mental disorder are more likely than others to be seeking a spiritual understanding of life. He writes: 'There is something at the core of the experience of mental illness that draws sufferers towards the spiritual. Their suffering is an echo of the suffering we all contain within us' (Razzaque, 2014: p. 5).

This issue comes to the fore when we consider how to respond to a person who is in need of psychiatric help and in the throes of a spiritual crisis, be it loss of faith or an experience of overwhelming spiritual significance. Mental health services provide little by way of spiritually informed care. Consequently, there is no way of knowing how often a transient psychotic episode might otherwise have become the turning point on a new path of meaning and purpose had the narrative only been explored in a different way.

This is a difficult area, especially as psychiatrists have a medically sanctioned role to relieve symptoms. It is neither their job to proselytise, nor is it their job to presume the role of spiritual advisor. Even so, by routinely taking a short spiritual history (Eagger, 2009), serious misunderstandings can be avoided. The Royal College of Psychiatrists has now affirmed that 'a tactful and sensitive exploration of patients' religious beliefs and spirituality should routinely be considered and will sometimes be an essential component of clinical assessment' (Cook, 2013).

The discussion that takes place between patient and psychiatrist is potentially one of the most intimate the patient will ever have. Yet the more the narrative adheres to the medical diagnostic approach, the less will the dialogue engage with real existential concerns. Rather than dive too deep, many psychiatrists argue that what appear to be tangled preoccupations with the self, the world and even the cosmos fade away on recovery, suggesting that the perplexity and ruminations were secondary to mental disorder – and therefore best left well alone.

At the same time, psychiatrists know that conflict, loss and soul-searching are implicated in most mental breakdowns. Body, mind and soul, whose interweaving remains the greatest conundrum in psychiatry, have to be taken together if the psychiatrist is to help the patient recover from breakdown to wholeness of being.

## Where the narratives of science and spirituality meet

Classical science regards consciousness and its spiritual *essentia* (the soul) as epiphenomena, arising (somehow) from the physico-chemical processes of the brain. This approach, derived from Newtonian mechanics,[1] treats the mind and its contents purely as emergent psychological phenomena (God included).

Such a physicalist approach is founded on study (and measurement) of the object. Because consciousness is experienced subjectively, it has therefore to be ruled out of court. Yet one thing everyone agrees on is that they are conscious! It seems that degrees of consciousness are present in all life forms, most probably in proportion to the complexity of neural structure. A cat or dog, for instance, has awareness similar to our own. But we humans have further evolved the capacity to be self-aware which, coupled with language, enables inner dialogue, personal history and identity, and freedom of choice.

The time-honoured metaphysical view, of which natural science has always been so intolerant, is now being reframed by the 'new' science of

---

1. Isaac Newton was himself deeply religious and saw no contradiction between his laws of physics and a creator God. He wrote, 'the motions which the planets now have could not spring from any natural cause alone, but were impressed by an intelligent Agent [...] not blind and fortuitous, but very well skilled in Mechanicks and Geometry' (Heller, 2009: p. 148).

quantum field theory, which seeks to understand the experimentally proven non-local properties of consciousness (Hameroff & Chopra, 2012). This perspective regards consciousness as pre-existent and pre-eminent; the brain as the on-board computer taps into a ubiquitous field of consciousness rather like a television picking up a broadcast signal and integrates it with the memory store of each person's experiences. The result: a unique and personal self-aware narrative.

The implications of these two perspectives are very different. The 'bottom-up' physicalist view sees each human being as a discrete entity, having an inner world composed only of personal experience and communicating with others solely by means of the special sense organs. On this basis, rationalists argue that God is nothing but a mental projection, good for warding off the (ego's) fear of oblivion and death.

The 'top-down' metaphysical view, on the other hand, sees every human being as participating in a shared consciousness that ultimately extends beyond the self, indeed beyond the bounds of individual birth and death. This approach is consonant with the proposition first made by Aristotle in *Metaphysics* that the whole is more than the sum of its parts; it opens the way to a fundamental figure/ground reversal so that 'God', far from being a mere projection, is the *materium primum* of all that is.

Must we choose either one or other narrative? Surely there is room for both, for the greater does not exclude the lesser. The physicist Thomas Campbell reminds us that the subsystem, in this case human intelligence, can never fully comprehend the system of which it is a part – what he calls the larger consciousness system (Campbell, 2007). Campbell uses the impartial language of physics when speaking of the data stream that conjoins part and whole. Yet in the subjective language of spirituality we find the same mystery in the powerful recognition that 'I belong to more than myself'.

The various faith traditions each frame this mystery in their own way. For example, while Islam deliberately refrains from representational images of Allah, the Judeo-Christian faiths envision God according to an archetypal Imago Dei. Hinduism has something of both; Brahman the supreme power cannot be described but manifests through a multitude of lesser deities. Buddhists eschew a personal God altogether. The burgeoning 'spiritual but not religious' demographic is more likely to speak of a unitive and all-embracing 'higher power' or 'ultimate truth'.

## Narratives of the soul

What, then, of the soul – a word notably absent from the vocabulary of psychiatry and strangely perhaps, given that *psyche* in Greek means soul? The soul does not have to imply transcendence; some will refer simply to what is best in humanity – compassion, wisdom, unconditional love and innate goodness. In this sense, everyone can be said to have a soul.

Others will regard the soul as the expression of the divine in human form – that we are souls and that this is the source of our capacity for love and our awareness of goodness, beauty and truth. To borrow from Pierre Teilhard de Chardin (2008), the difference in perspective is whether we see ourselves as human beings on a spiritual journey or spiritual beings on a human journey.

Either way, the human soul escapes any narrow definition and yet it holds a sacred meaning for all creeds and cultures. As Carl Jung pointed out, the soul is an archetype with profound symbolism second only to the supreme archetype of the Imago Dei (Jung, 1951).

From the standpoint of enabling patients to come from the deepest place within, psychiatrists need to accept that words such as 'God' and 'soul' are for some people instinctive and necessary when questioning the meaning and purpose of human existence, and what may lie beyond the physical bounds of birth and death. The psychiatrist simply needs to stay open-minded and be genuinely interested in where the spiritual narrative leads.

The psychiatric assessment, not least the mental state examination, is necessarily structured and formal to a degree. Even so, once the patient's welfare and safety is assured and the necessary treatment measures are put in place, there is the opportunity for a different kind of heartfelt narrative to unfold. For the psychiatrist, this entails suspending judgement and engaging compassionately with one's patient as a fellow human being. It means being willing to 'accompany' the patient in searching for answers to the big questions of life and death, including the nature and purpose of the soul, while trusting that the mental health crisis, however painful, can lead to an enrichment of life and its values, sometimes with new and very different life goals (Powell, 2009).

Much of this is what good counselling and psychotherapy offers – empathy, warmth and genuineness, as researched nearly 50 years ago by Truax & Carkhuff (1967). But here the psychiatrist ventures further. Spirituality has two dimensions: the quest for answers to the ultimate meaning and purpose of life, and the experience of wholeness of being that can bring inner strength and peace. By supporting a soulful narrative, the psychiatrist helps those profound questions to be asked perhaps for the first time (Spirituality and Psychiatry Special Interest Group, 2014). Then, as with the proverb of the person who is searching everywhere until they realise the necklace is already around their neck, the patient who begins to find their own answers to those deep questions discovers a wisdom they never knew they had and one that can help bring peace of mind.

Such conversations are, in fact, conversations 'soul-to-soul'. Whatever arises will happen naturally and exactly as it should when the psychiatrist is able to be fully 'present' and concerned only to help the patient find his or her 'truth'.

The soul narrative can often be elicited with a few simple prompts. Sometimes it helps to amplify what a patient has begun to say or to encourage a person to think the 'unthinkable'. For instance, if someone is contemplating suicide, it is worth finding out whether they believe death is the absolute and final end. If the patient is unsure (as many are), it makes sense to ask 'If there were to be an existence or a world beyond, how would you imagine it to be?' Encouragement to step outside the life being lived can bring a different perspective to bear, one that is wiser, more forgiving and more compassionate than the harsh self-judgement that so often accompanies mental anguish, as the following example shows:

> A young man burdened with a deep sense of failure and unable to see any future found himself in fear and trembling before God. Invited to 'listen' to what God might say to him, to his surprise he found himself being gently admonished, then lovingly told to continue with his life and to remember that success is not measured by wealth or fame but by finding love for his friends, his family and himself.

In cases of traumatic bereavement, the psychiatrist can ask about things left unresolved or unsaid that might be important to address. Often the patient will begin by saying it is too late. Instead, they can be invited to close their eyes, form a picture of the loved one and speak to them as if they were right there in the room. Not only can what was unexpressed now be voiced, but a narrative of healing can begin. By guiding the patient into a conversation (e.g. 'What do you need to ask/tell the person?' followed by 'Now listen to what they need to say to you') the soul can make itself heard, as shown in this example:

> A middle-aged woman had cared for her ageing father during his final illness and decline. Although close, their relationship had often been a tense one, and as he became more infirm and fought his disability, she often felt he was fighting her too. At times she got frustrated and angry, and then guilty for having such feelings. After her father passed away, she became depressed, reproaching herself for not 'having done better'. Assisted by the psychiatrist, she was able to 'meet' her father. She was encouraged to tell him about feeling how she had let him down. To her surprise, the answer came back that he was deeply grateful for the help and support she had given. He 'said' to her, 'I know you did your very best. I am grateful, I love you and I want you to be happy'. The daughter and father could now part with a loving farewell.

Often problems that might seem insoluble can be approached by 'going within' and listening to the soul directly:

> A man brought up alone by an abusive alcoholic mother was suffering from chronic depression, heavily laced with anger towards his mother. He could see that bitterness was spoiling his life but could only bring himself to say 'I'll never forgive what she did to me'. The therapist asked him if he *wished* that he could forgive. He replied, 'more than anything but it's impossible'. The psychiatrist now knew that although the egoic mind would not relent, the soul's capacity for forgiveness was present, so she invited him to 'go within' and find out what his heart would say if it could only speak.[2] His heart said to him, 'I am

---

2. *Le cœur a ses raisons, que la raison ne connaît point* [The heart has its reasons, which reason does not know] (Pascal, 1660).

in such pain. All this anger is hurting me. Please stop before I break. I'm here to bring love into your life. Don't turn your back on me'. The patient fell silent for a while, sighed and then said, to himself as much as the psychiatrist, 'It's time I stopped hating and started loving. I want to get a life while there's time'.

## In conclusion

I have set out to show how, across a wide range of clinical objectives, paying attention to narrative is important both for diagnosis and for treatment. Starting with the physical, I describe how narrative changes when engaging with the mental, and how making sense of the patient's story becomes a co-creation of doctor and patient. Lastly, I explore how narrative changes yet again when the focus moves to the spiritual.

This further shift is a profound one, for the narrative of the soul knows no bounds. Transcending the limitations of the mundane life, soul wisdom brings a deeper understanding to the human predicament. When the psychiatrist is willing to be fully 'present', and able to offer a genuine and heartfelt connection with the individual who is in pain, the way is opened to reconciliation, forgiveness and peace of mind. The key lies in this: though the ego may be deeply aggrieved, the soul always seeks to love. The psychiatrist who can reach out to the soul in their patient is privileged to share in a narrative that brings healing to the psyche and fresh hope to the dispirited.

## References

Campbell, T. (2007) *My Big Toe: A Trilogy Unifying Philosophy, Physics, and Metaphysics: Awakening, Discovery, Inner Workings*. Lightning Strike Books.

Cook, C.C.H. (2013) *Recommendations for Psychiatrists on Spirituality and Religion* (Position Statement PS03/2013). Royal College of Psychiatrists.

Cook, C.C.H. & Powell, A. (2013) Spirituality is not bad for our mental health. *British Journal of Psychiatry*, **202**, 385–6.

Cox, M. (1982) 'I took a life because I needed one': psychotherapeutic possibilities with the schizophrenic offender-patient. *Psychotherapy and Psychosomatics*, **37**, 96–105.

Davies, J. (2013) *Cracked: Why Psychiatry is Doing More Harm Than Good*. Icon Books.

De Waal, M., Arnold, I., Eekhof, J., et al (2004) Somatoform disorders in general practice: prevalence, functional impairment and comorbidity with anxiety and depressive disorders. *British Journal of Psychiatry*, **184**, 470–6.

Eagger, S. (2009) A guide to the assessment of spiritual concerns in mental healthcare. Royal College of Psychiatrists. Available at http://www.rcpsych.ac.uk/pdf/A_guide_to_the_assessment_of_spiritual_concerns_in_mental_healthcare.pdf (accessed 5 November 2015).

Farooq, S. (2012) Is acute and transient psychotic disorder (ATPD) mini schizophrenia? The evidence from phenomenology and epidemiology. *Psychiatria Danubina*, **24** (suppl. 3), 311–5.

Fitzgerald, E. (1859) (transl.) *The Rubáiyát of Omar Khayyám*. Collins, 1989.

Freud, S. (1937) Analysis terminable and interminable. In *The Standard Edition of the Complete Psychological Works of Sigmund Freud*. Volume 23. Hogarth Press, 1968.

Hameroff, S. & Chopra, D. (2012) The 'Quantum Soul'. In *Exploring Frontiers of the Mind-Brain Relationship* (eds A. Moreira-Almeida, F. Santana Santos). Springer.

Heller, M. (2009) *Ultimate Explanations of the Universe*. Springer.
Herrigel, E. (1953) *Zen in the Art of Archery*. Routledge and Kegan Paul.
Ilibagiza, I. (2006) *Left To Tell*. Hay House.
Jung, C. (1951) Researches into the phenomenology of the self. In *Collected Works*. Vol. 9, Part 2: Aion. Routledge and Kegan Paul.
King M., Marston L., McManus S., et al (2013) Religion, spirituality and mental health: results from a national study of English households. *British Journal of Psychiatry*, **202**, 68–73.
Koenig, H.G., King, D.E. & Carson, V.B. (2012) *Handbook of Religion and Health*, 2nd edn. Oxford University Press.
Lucas, C. (2011) *In Case Of Spiritual Emergency*. Findhorn Press.
Mental Health Foundation (n.d.) Mental health statistics. Available at http://www.mentalhealth.org.uk/help-information/mental-health-statistics/ (accessed 5 November 2015).
Pargament, K.I. (2011) *Spiritually Integrated Psychotherapy: Understanding and Addressing the Sacred*. Guilford Press.
Pascal, B. (1660) *Pensees*. Transl. W.F. Trotter. Section IV: 'Of the Means of Belief': p. 277. Reprinted: 2005. Digireads.com.
Powell, A. (2009) Soul-centred psychotherapy. Available at http://www.rcpsych.ac.uk/college/specialinterestgroups/spirituality/publications.aspx#p (accessed 5 November 2015).
Powell, A. (2013) Modernity and the beleaguered soul. Available at http://www.rcpsych.ac.uk/college/specialinterestgroups/spirituality/publications.aspx#p (accessed on 5 November 2015).
Queirazza, F., Semple, D.M. & Lawrie, S.M. (2014) Transition to schizophrenia in acute and transient psychotic disorders. *British Journal of Psychiatry*, **204**, 299–305.
Razzaque, R. (2014) *Breaking Down Is Waking Up*. Watkins Publishing.
Rogers, C. (1961) *On Becoming a Person: A Therapist's View of Psychotherapy*. Houghton Mifflin.
Romme, M. & Escher, A. (1989) Hearing voices. *Schizophrenia Bulletin*, **15**, 209–16.
Scheeres, J. (2011) *A Thousand Lives: The Untold Story of Jonestown*. Simon & Schuster.
Shorter, E. (2014) The 25th anniversary of the launch of Prozac gives pause for thought: where did we go wrong? *British Journal of Psychiatry*, **204**, 331–2.
Spirituality and Psychiatry Special Interest Group (2014) Spirituality and mental health ('Mental Health Information' leaflet). Royal College of Psychiatrists. Available at http://www.rcpsych.ac.uk/mentalhealthinformation/therapies/spiritualityandmentalhealth.aspx (accessed 5 November 2015).
Summerville, C. (2009) Your recovery journey. Available at http://www.your-recovery-journey.ca/Message.htm (accessed 5 November 2015).
Szasz, T. (1960) The myth of mental illness. *American Psychologist*, **15**, 113–18.
Teilhard de Chardin, P. (2008) *The Phenomenon of Man*. Harper Perennial.
Truax, C.B. & Carkhuff, R.R. (1967) *Towards Effective Counseling and Psychotherapy*. Aldine.
Williams, R. (2011) How the drug companies are controlling our lives. *Psychology Today*, 13 May. Available at http://www.psychologytoday.com/blog/wired-success/201105/how-the-drug-companies-are-controlling-our-lives-part-1 (accessed 5 November 2015).
World Health Organization (n.d.) Global burden of disease. Available at http://www.who.int/healthinfo/global_burden_disease/gbd/en/ (accessed 5 November 2015).
World Health Organization (2016) *International Statistical Classification of Diseases and Related Health Problems, 10th Revision (ICD-10)*. Version: 2016. WHO. Available at: http://apps.who.int/classifications/icd10/browse/2016/en (accessed 27 January 2016).

CHAPTER 5

# Gods lost and found: spiritual coping in clinical practice

James Lomax and Kenneth I. Pargament

Historically, religion and spirituality have not been treated particularly kindly by mental health practitioners and theorists, being described as passive and defensive in character and oriented towards denying rather than confronting the realities of life (Pargament & Park, 1995). Albert Ellis, the founder of rational emotive therapy, had this to say: 'the conclusion seems inescapable that religiosity is, on almost every conceivable count, opposed to the normal goals of mental health' (1986: p. 42). In the past 25 years this critical view has given way to a more balanced perspective. Ellis himself recanted his uniformly negative stance. The shift in view may be in part due to the emergence of a significant body of empirical research linking religion and spirituality to better health and well-being in many groups, including clinical populations (Koenig *et al*, 2012).

This chapter focuses on one significant domain of research and its implications for clinical practice: the cognitive and relational domains of spiritual coping. We begin with a brief review of theory and research in the area of spiritual coping, particularly as it applies to people dealing with mental health problems (for more comprehensive reviews see Cummings & Pargament, 2010; Pargament, 2011; Gall & Guirguis-Younger, 2013). We then present two narrative accounts of spiritual coping in clinical practice, which illustrate different patterns of spiritual coping and different directions in treatment. We conclude by considering ways to foster greater sensitivity among mental health professionals to the important place of spirituality in treatment.

## Theory and research on spiritual coping

### Prevalence of spiritual coping

The adage that there are no atheists in foxholes is not wholly correct. Even in an event as horrific as the Holocaust, some people reported themselves to be non-believers before, during and well after this trauma (Brenner, 1980). Yet, though it is not a universal rule, the spiritual impulse is often quickened during times of greatest stress. This holds true not only for the general population but also for people with serious psychiatric problems. In one study, 30% of patients described an increase in their religious faith following the development of a psychiatric illness (Kirov *et al*, 1998). In another study of 400 out-patients with serious mental illness, 80% reported that they used religion to cope. Moreover, almost half of their total coping time was devoted to religious activities (Tepper *et al*, 2001). Psychiatric patients may be even more likely to draw on religious beliefs and practices in coping than the general population (Neeleman & Lewis, 1994). It appears that many people with significant mental health problems turn to their faith in difficult times. To what end?

## *The functions of spiritual coping*

Theorists have long debated the purposes served by religion and spirituality (see Pargament, 2013 for review). Freud saw religion as rooted in two motivations: the need to control sexual and aggressive impulses and the need to allay the fears that accompany the confrontation with human frailty and finitude. Durkheim (1915) emphasized the role religion serves in fostering social bonds and identity. Similarly, theorists such as Lee Kirkpatrick (2005) and Jon Allen (2013) have underscored the part that religion and spirituality can play in facilitating connectedness that provides individuals with both a safe harbour and a secure base for exploration of the world. Anthropologist Clifford Geertz (1966), psychiatrist Viktor Frankl (1984) and more recently, psychologist Crystal Park (2013) have each addressed the ways in which religion and spirituality provide people with a way to make meaning of seemingly nonsensical events. Others have described how religion and spirituality work to promote self-development, personal transformation and evolutionary advantage.

There is empirical evidence to support many of these perspectives. For example, consistent with the assertion that religion serves the purposes of impulse control and self-regulation, higher levels of religiousness and spirituality have been consistently tied to lower levels of substance use, crime and delinquency, and greater conscientiousness (McCullough & Carter, 2013). Consistent with attachment theory, a number of studies have demonstrated how beliefs in God can function as sources of secure attachment and compensations for deficits in attachments with parents (Granqvist & Kirkpatrick, 2013).

Studies such as these suggest that religion and spirituality may serve multiple purposes. Part of the staying power of religion and spirituality may lie in their ability to meet the diverse needs of different people. A study of 115 Swiss out-patients with schizophrenia or schizoaffective disorder addresses this (Mohr *et al*, 2006). The researchers interviewed the patients about their spiritual beliefs and practices and the roles they serve in their daily lives and in coping with their illness and its consequences. The interviews were then content analysed. Patients described a wide range of functions that spiritual coping resources played in their lives: comfort, meaning-making, hope, self-respect and self-confidence, compassion, love and enjoyment of life.

In discussing the psychological and social functions of spiritual coping, it is important to avoid the dangers of radical reductionism, that is, explaining religion and spirituality away as merely expressions of deeper underlying of psychological and social motivations. To the spiritually minded, including spiritually minded patients, religion and spirituality are ends in themselves. As psychologist of religion Paul Johnson put it: 'It is the ultimate thou that the religious person seeks most of all' (1959: p. 70). Theorists have also suggested that religious and spiritual motivations can become 'functionally autonomous' of more basic drives or primary motivations in and of themselves (see Pargament, 2013). Additional research is needed to determine whether spirituality represents a distinctive motivation. Nevertheless, practitioners should be aware that many people, including patients, experience their faith as a central, organizing and motivating force in their lives. Caution is needed, then, when religious and spiritual beliefs and practices are interpreted in terms of presumably deeper motivations.

## The many methods of spiritual coping

Given the purposes it may serve, it is not surprising that spirituality can express itself in many ways when people face traumatic events. The religions of the world have provided their adherents with a number of methods of dealing with major stressors (Box 5.1). In contrast to stereotypes about religion, these coping methods are generally more active than passive. As one survivor of clergy sexual abuse put it: 'I think I have matured – I have developed a belief that God may not take care of me the way I like, he does not swoop down and fix things even when we are praying, but he can take our brokenness and create strength' (Murray-Swank & Waelde, 2013: p. 338).

Empirical studies have shown that spiritual coping methods are associated with positive mental health outcomes among non-clinical and clinical samples. For example, in Mohr's study of patients with schizophrenia and schizoaffective disorders, positive spiritual coping was predictive of more favourable outcomes 3 years later with respect to negative symptoms, social adaptation and quality of life (Mohr *et al*, 2011). In another prospective study of psychotic patients in partial day treatment, positive religious coping was tied to improvement in depression, anxiety and psychological well-being, accounting for 25%, 35% and 24% of the changes on these outcomes respectively (Rosmarin *et al*, 2013). These findings suggest that spiritual coping methods can be a significant resource for many patients in treatment.

## Spiritual struggles

There is, however, a darker potential outcome of spiritual and religious resources. Major life events, including serious mental illness, can shake

> **Box 5.1** Definitions and indicators of religious and spiritual coping methods and struggles
>
> Positive religious and spiritual coping methods
>
> - **Benevolent religious reappraisal** – redefining the stressor through religion as potentially beneficial ('I try to see how God might be trying to strengthen me in this situation')
> - **Collaborative religious coping** – seeking control through a partnership with God in problem-solving ('I look to God for strength, support, and guidance')
> - **Active religious surrender** – active giving up of control to God in coping ('I try to do the best I can and let God do the rest')
> - **Religious purification** – searching for spiritual cleansing through religious actions ('I ask forgiveness for my sins')
> - **Spiritual connection** – seeking a sense of connectedness with forces that transcend the self ('I try to build a strong relationship with a higher power')
> - **Seeking support from clergy or members** – searching for intimacy and reassurance through the life and care of congregation members and clergy ('I ask others to pray for me')
> - **Religious helping** – attempting to provide spiritual support and comfort to others ('I try to provide others with spiritual comfort')
> - **Seeking religious direction** – looking to religion for assistance in finding a new direction for living ('I look to God for a new direction in life')
>
> Religious and spiritual struggles[1]
>
> - **Struggles with the divine** – experiencing feelings of anger towards, abandonment by, or being punished by, God ('I feel angry at God')
> - **Struggles with the demonic** – experiencing feelings of being attacked, possessed or punished by the Devil ('I feel attacked by the Devil or by evil spirits')
> - **Interpersonal struggles** – conflicts, disagreements or tensions with other people about religious and spiritual matters ('I feel angry at organized religion')
> - **Doubt-related struggles** – questioning religious beliefs and practices ('I feel confused about my religious/spiritual beliefs')
> - **Moral struggles** – experiencing guilt and shame about failures to live up to moral standards and religious values ('I worry that my actions are morally or spiritually wrong')
> - **Struggles of ultimate meaning** – questioning the ultimate meaning and purpose of one's life ('I question whether life really matters')
>
> 1. Source: Exline *et al*, 2014.

or shatter people spiritually as well as emotionally, socially and physically. Several studies have highlighted the negative impact of sexual trauma and abuse on spirituality as manifested by declines in loving images of God, the sense of spiritual well-being, involvement in institutional religious life, and increases in feelings of being punished or abandoned by God (Murray-Swank & Waelde, 2013). Working with a group of war veterans who were being treated for post-traumatic stress disorder, Fontana & Rosenheck

(2004) reported that the experiences of witnessing or participating in the killing of others weakened religious faith.

Researchers have begun to focus their attention on one type of spiritual problem in particular – spiritual struggles. Spiritual struggles have been defined as tension, strain and conflict about spiritual matters within oneself (intrapsychic), with others (interpersonal) and with the Divine (supernatural) (Pargament *et al*, 2005; Exline, 2013). More specific forms of spiritual struggle have also been delineated and assessed, as shown in Box 5.1 (Exline *et al*, 2014). Struggles of these kinds, while less frequent than positive spiritual coping, are not rare: 62% of a national sample reported that they were sometimes angry at God (Exline *et al*, 2011). According to the 1999 General Social Survey, 23.2% of a national sample reported that they feel God may be punishing them and 12% reported wondering whether God had abandoned them (Fetzer Institute & National Institute on Aging Working Group, 1999). Spiritual struggles appear to be an outgrowth of both situational and personality factors. In this vein, Ano & Pargament (2012) found that spiritual struggles were more likely to be experienced by people dealing with more serious life stressors, an insecure ambivalent attachment to God and higher levels of neuroticism.

Spiritual struggles have also been robustly associated with poorer mental health and physical health. In a large national survey, McConnell and colleagues (2006) reported that spiritual struggles were linked with a variety of measures of psychopathology, including depression, anxiety, paranoid ideation and somatization. Spiritual struggles have also been associated with poorer functioning among several psychiatric samples (see Exline, 2013 for a review). For example, in a longitudinal study of 48 young adults diagnosed with schizophrenia or bipolar disorder, those who reported more divine struggles in relationship to their illness manifested increases in psychiatric symptoms over 1 year (Phillips & Stein, 2007). These findings have been extended to non-Christian samples, including Jews, Muslims, Hindus and Buddhists (Abu-Raiya & Pargament, 2015). Finally, a few studies have suggested that people who experience chronic or unresolved spiritual struggles are at greater risk for subsequent psychological and physical problems (Pargament *et al*, 2004).

## From research to practice: two clinical narratives

Although empirical research has shown important links between spirituality and health and well-being, practitioners have only just begun to address spirituality in the context of clinical treatment. Given the sensitivity of the topic, it is important to approach spirituality carefully. In this regard, narrative accounts can play an important role in facilitating spiritually sensitive mental health training and treatment (e.g. Lomax *et al*, 2011).

Even though concerns about religious and spiritual issues may lead patients to seek help from religious officials, these concerns are less commonly reasons for consultation with mental health professionals. While spiritual struggles do produce overt psychopathology such as depression, anxiety, panic or substance misuse, they are often overshadowed by the psychiatric problems (clinical symptoms) that the patient discusses initially. Only later is it sometimes evident that a spiritual struggle has been a significant preceding factor. The following vignettes (the narratives of Sylvia and Arnold) are illustrative of two different patterns of spiritual struggle, coping and approaches to treatment.

## *Narrative 1. Sylvia*

Sylvia was an early career paediatric hospital physician referred by her clinical unit director because her irritability and uncooperativeness had interfered with the functioning of her team. Her performance was especially surprising given her prior academic excellence and personal history of community service. At our first meeting, she clearly met criteria for mild to moderate major depression. As part of routine questioning, I asked about her use of religious or spiritual coping. She angrily snapped 'I knew you were going to ask about that. It's none of your business, and I don't want someone telling me to go to Sunday school'. I asked how she was so certain that I was going to bring up religion. She said she had 'googled' me after I was recommended by her 'sanctimonious service chief'. She had seen that I had written 'a bunch of religious crap' but had not read any of it 'because that would have been snooping'.

I was a bit surprised, but managed to say it sounded like she was feeling pretty desperate and trying to figure out what sort of partner I might be for an important project. We spent the rest of our first meeting discussing a trial of a selective serotonin reuptake inhibitor (SSRI) to help manage her symptoms.

Over the next few weeks her symptoms slowly began to attenuate and we agreed that I would get to know her better by taking a developmental history. Of particular relevance is that she was the eldest child of a career military father, reared with expectations of 'following orders', and influenced by his opinion that 'good thoughts produce good deeds and a good life' when lived out in a 'solid faith community'. Influenced by the work of Ana-Maria Rizutto (1979), I wondered about my patient's intrapsychic connection of God and father images and the implication of that connection for other attachment relationships, but initially focused on symptom reduction and developing a therapeutic alliance.

About 3 months into our relationship, her symptoms of depression were much improved. I felt able to ask her if she had any further reflections on our rocky start when I had asked her about her religious and spiritual life. This exchange was quite different from my first attempt. It seemed that her father was quite pleased when she first mentioned applying to medical school. In fact, he was excited and 'sure' that she would want to be a medical missionary in their faith tradition, serving as 'a soldier like him' but fighting a different sort of 'crusade'. For a while, Sylvia had considered a career in mission work but later developed academic aspirations. She thought a compromise might be found in providing education and service within paediatric intensive care units. Her father seemed a bit disappointed, but accepting of her change.

However, something unexpected happened within her as she repeatedly watched innocent children die from horrible illnesses, and medical treatments that 'produced more suffering than cure'. This change was greatly accelerated during her treatment of 'Paul', an adorable 6-year-old with advanced neuroblastoma. His last 6 months included four 'miserable' hospitalizations under her care. She remembered his last night tearfully and her angry declaration that 'no loving God could let something like this happen'. She felt deceived by both her father and her God. We began to wonder whether her disappointments might have also been expressed by her generalized surliness, her lack of cooperativeness with colleagues and her harshness with students.

About 6 months into our work, her cognitive and vegetative symptoms of depression were attenuated, but she wondered about a feeling that there was 'something missing' in her life. She reported that she had left the faith community of her childhood while her symptoms had been increasing. She wondered if that community was part of what was missing, but quickly added that she could not return to a belief system that produced so much guilt when 'bad things happen to good people'.

She went on to report the 'silly idea' of exploring a very different faith community, but was aware she was afraid of mentioning that to me. She said that when she thought about doing so, she imagined me saying she was 'wishy-washy and waffling'. I expressed my concern that 'the shadow of your little girl relationship with your father makes some paths hard to explore' in our project. She smiled and mentioned a particular faith community she had considered based on comments of a friend. She did not know much about their beliefs except that they were very different from those of her childhood. She wondered if she would have to believe exactly like them in order to be welcomed. Fortuitously, I happened to know the leader of that community and asked if she had considered arranging a meeting with him to have that discussion. She said she would do that but quickly admonished me not to speak to him and observed that I seemed 'more directive' than usual.

Of course, I was concerned about what would happen, and also about my boundary crossing. I was quite relieved when she reported on the discussion. They had talked about the value of spiritual community as a separate dimension from particular religious beliefs. My acquaintance had also suggested a book by a different faith leader that described a theology without the linear relationships between ideas or feelings and outcomes that had led to her traumatic disillusionment in life – accompanied by irritable depression and isolation (Karff, 2005). She also mentioned how 'silly' she felt at the first service when she had no idea what the cantor was singing about, but how his voice and the music brought tears and relief. I responded that I wouldn't be much help about the ideas or beliefs of the cantor, but finding some intimation of a sacred community seemed more like an important achievement than 'something silly'.

## Interpretation

Sylvia's depression emerged from the combination of multiple tragic losses of children she felt called to care for and a spiritual struggle arising from a traumatic disillusionment with her psychological construct of the God, who she felt had called her to provide that care. Initially she had great reluctance to share her religious and spiritual experiences, including her doubts or her loss of community. Her God image was heavily influenced by her childhood perception of her father, and his assertion that adversity was given to us as a sort of test of our will and ability to pursue challenges as 'God's soldiers' (or doctors). She was afraid to question those in authority and became progressively angrier when her efforts did not produce the outcomes she sought to achieve.

In a therapeutic transference relationship she anxiously experimented with whether a new attachment figure would expect only rigid obedience and disciplined rule-following. She wondered whether I could appreciate her experiences and doubts – especially doubts about any 'plans' I might have for her. As I, imperfectly but adequately enough, passed these tests she felt more freedom to explore a wider range of her own ideas, feelings and uncertainties. Questioning my intentions and plans was frightening, but her success in the practice field of our relationship led not only to a novel feeling of safety in the therapeutic relationship but also to a realization that she had frequently assumed that a variety of authority figures had been critical of her, leaving her feeling angry and isolated because of those assumptions.

As a correlate of this freedom, Sylvia slowly became more aware of her relatively unexamined internal life, including her spiritual struggles (making its unconscious content conscious) and becoming more accepting of human imperfections in herself and others. She initially used her exploratory psychodynamic psychotherapy to make connections between a spectrum of relationships in which she felt anger and tension.

Her presenting symptoms attenuated but she still felt that something was missing. Beginning within the therapeutic relationship, she began to nurture the ability to be more curious about not only herself but also those in her environment with different ideas and values. She was eventually able to explore and make a connection to a faith community that was a better fit for her and her adult life experiences. Her participation in a new faith community was not an easy transition for her family. However, they had been aware of how miserable she had been and eventually accepted that 'at least she had found some sort of religious home'.

## Narrative 2. Arnold

> Arnold is a 64-year-old labourer, whose wife developed rapidly progressive Alzheimer's disease a year before their long-anticipated retirement. He was seen by the psychiatrist member of an Alzheimer's Caregivers team following comments he made to the effect that he would have better times together with his wife in the near future, hinting at suicidal plans. As his wife's memory and orientation difficulties escalated, Arnold said he could feel the future they had planned slipping away. He was furious and depressed about the 'unfairness' of these events. In an effort to find solace, he had switched from a conservative, non-denominational church to worshipping as a Jehovah's Witness. In this new religious participation, he 'knew God's name as Jehovah for the first time'. He found his solace in the 'promised New Order to come', in which good and decent people like him and his wife would be restored and rewarded, and the wicked would be punished. He also found himself welcomed into a community that provided both a caring interest in his situation and practical support for his family.

The specifics of Arnold's faith community were not well known to the therapist and the therapeutic activity was mostly active listening and supporting Arnold's ideas that involved positive religious coping (God loved him and wanted good things for him and his wife) and healthy religious activity (Arnold's role as a teacher in his faith community as a generative activity). Interventions were largely clarification without significant interpretation of either defensive ideas or the displaced and sublimated aggression involved in the New Order. Arnold seemed convinced that the New Order would be a time for him and his wife to enjoy the good experiences they had earned. Furthermore, in the New Order, evil people who had seemed to 'get away with' their bad behaviour would have a much more enduring period of suffering than they had experienced in human or earthly time. In this New Order, he and his wife would be valued and appreciated partners of God.

## Interpretation

Like Sylvia, Arnold experienced life challenges that threw him into spiritual struggle. His wife's dementia represented a profound threat to his most fundamental beliefs in ultimate justice and compensation in this world. These struggles were accompanied by depression and rage. Arnold sought out a new religious direction and religious conversion to cope with his struggles. His change in religious identification and participation was highly dependent on specific religious cognitions that allowed him to hold on to his beliefs in ultimate justice, an ultimate reunion with his wife, and an ultimate loving God.

His religious participation could be regarded as defensive, both psychologically (rationalization and reaction-formation in his attitude towards God) and theologically (the need to envisage a just fate for the wicked in order to preserve the contrasting thought of a loving and rewarding God). However, it was also adaptive, producing hope, shared beliefs, and a community in which he both received help and was able to help other caregivers. The shared beliefs functioned as creative illusions (Meissner, 1984) that reflected the inner significance of a new, highly specific belief system shared by a socially active and involved community. There was a health-promoting synergy between Arnold's beliefs and his faith community, where he was chosen to be an Elder. This allowed him to serve as a teacher and leader and gave significance to his current life, which was especially important because he had lost the long-treasured retirement years of travel and co-grandparenting he had planned with his wife. His role in his faith community provided much needed compensation for the unexpected loneliness and loss of the companionship he had anticipated sharing with his wife.

In the case of Arnold, exploring the defensive aspects of his religious beliefs and conversion to Jehovah's Witness seemed ill-advised on several accounts. His beliefs were not only egosyntonic, they were also affirmed by a community in which he was valued. The group members shared a vision of God in which he and the group not only 'knew God's name', but also felt known and to-be-rewarded by God in God's time. Arnold's religious cognitions did not produce distress and a therapeutic alliance to address them was not, therefore, feasible. Instead, supportive psychotherapy helped Arnold to use his beliefs to suppress certain emotions such as anger at earthly injustices that might otherwise have been mobilized in ways that were unlikely to be beneficial.

Arnold's treatment was intermittently challenging for the therapist since his vision for the New Order was at great variance with his therapist's values. In one way psychotherapy with Arnold was fairly simple – it was easy to be curious about his faith community and his role in it. This was especially true with how Arnold found meaning and meaningfulness in his generative actions as a teacher and leader in his community. Supporting generativity is probably health-promoting as well as correlated with 'aging well' (Vaillant, 2002). However, at other times, Arnold's religious beliefs created countertransference challenges. His religious beliefs and vision of the afterlife included intensely dichotomous outcomes for people based on their adherence to narrowly defined religiosity and behaviour. For some therapists, religious beliefs about evil expressed as racial prejudices or highly discriminatory beliefs about differences in sexual orientation can create significant countertransference distancing or even dismissiveness and expressions of disapproval that challenge the therapeutic alliance. Although the therapist will often be able to deflect or attempt to extinguish hateful comments by neglecting them, Arnold's passionate disapproval of 'niggers and queers' generated strong negative countertransference responses in his therapist.

## Conclusions and recommendations

Working with spiritual issues in treatment calls for the same basic clinical skills needed for all therapeutic practice – sensitivity, openness and empathy. In this sense, spiritually sensitive care is not a brand new form of treatment (Pargament, 2007). Neither is it a competitor to established therapeutic orientations such as psychodynamic, cognitive–behavioural, dialectical-behavioural, and acceptance and commitment therapies. Instead, it involves the thoughtful integration of the spiritual dimension of the patient's life into treatment. As demonstrated in a growing body of theory and research, spirituality represents both a potential coping resource that can facilitate the health and well-being of patients and a potential source of struggle that can elicit, exacerbate or interfere with the resolution of psychiatric problems. It follows that a one-size-fits-all approach to psychiatric care is inappropriate for patients dealing with spiritual issues, just as it is for patients facing other concerns.

The two narratives presented in this chapter highlight how practitioners may address spiritual coping resources and spiritual struggles in clinical practice. In the case of Sylvia, exploratory psychotherapy was helpful in addressing spiritual struggles that were manifesting themselves through psychiatric symptomatology. Research on spiritual struggles has assumed that people have some degree of conscious awareness of their spiritual conflicts, tensions and strain; participants in research are asked to respond to items assessing various indicators of struggle. However, as the case of Sylvia shows, not all spiritual struggles are necessarily conscious. This should not be particularly surprising given the high level of distress that accompanies conflicts in the spiritual domain. As with other forms of deep conflict, practitioners can help their patients uncover core religious and spiritual tensions that may be expressed in psychological and physical problems. The practitioner's task is not to provide a theological resolution to these conflicts but to provide a safe, supportive context in which spiritual struggles can be understood, accepted and explored. This process may, in turn, have important psychiatric benefits for patients.

In other cases, such as that of Arnold, a supportive form of psychotherapy may help to encourage patients who are drawing on positive religious coping resources in the face of trauma and spiritual struggles. The practitioner does not have to be a theist or member of a religious community in order to appreciate and encourage patients who themselves believe in God or who participate in religious institutional life, traditional or non-traditional. Empirical studies have repeatedly pointed to the benefits of various religious and spiritual coping resources among people dealing with a full range of life challenges, including serious mental illness. This is not to say that certain religious and spiritual expressions cannot be potentially harmful. Clinical discernment in the area of spirituality is necessary in determining when various human thoughts and practices are harmful or helpful.

Cognitive–behavioural approaches may also be helpful when patients have become disconnected from religious and spiritual coping activities that could prove valuable to them as sources of support, meaning and hope in times of stress and struggle. Just as practitioners encourage their patients to access other resources in treatment (e.g. exercise, medication, social support), they can help patients identify and draw on latent religious and spiritual resources that may have been forgotten or neglected in the midst of psychiatric problems.

Practitioners are just beginning to attend to the spiritual dimension of patients' lives in treatment. For this nascent area of practice to advance further, several steps are needed. First, there is a need for more knowledge and understanding of spirituality – its multidimensional, multi-functional and dynamic character, and its double-sided capacity to both foster and impede health and well-being. Basic research is called for as well as applied clinical studies that examine the effectiveness of more spiritually sensitive and integrated treatments. Initial work in this area has yielded some promising results (e.g. Smith *et al*, 2007). Second, more training is sorely needed. Graduate training programmes in the mental health professions generally offer little or no training on religion and spirituality, leaving students ill-prepared to address the religious and spiritual issues they will encounter in their professional roles (e.g. Brawer *et al*, 2002). Finally, compelling clinical narratives of the kind presented in this volume are needed to help guide both researchers and clinicians interested in developing greater understanding and skills in this vital area of study and practice.

# References

Abu-Raiya, H. & Pargament, K.I. (2015) Religious coping among diverse religions: commonalities and divergences. *Psychology of Religion and Spirituality*, **7**, 24–33.

Allen, J.G. (2013) *Restoring Mentalizing in Attachment Relationships: Treating Trauma with Plain Old Therapy*. American Psychiatric Publishing.

Ano, G.G. & Pargament, K.I. (2012) Predictors of spiritual struggles: an exploratory study. *Mental Health, Religion and Culture*, **16**, 419–34.

Brawer, P.A., Handal, P.J., Fabricatore, A.N., *et al* (2002) Training and education in religion/spirituality within APA-accredited clinical psychology programs. *Professional Psychology: Research and Practice*, **33**, 203–6.

Brenner, R. (1980) *The Faith and Doubt of Holocaust Survivors*. Free Press.

Cummings, J.P. & Pargament, K.I. (2010) Medicine for the spirit: religious coping in individuals with medical conditions. *Religions*, **1**, 28–53.

Durkheim, E. (1915) *The Elementary Forms of the Religious Life*. Free Press. Available at http://www.gutenberg.org/ (accessed 23 February 2016).

Ellis, A. (1986) *The Case Against Religion: A Psychotherapist's View and the Case Against Religiosity*. American Atheist Press.

Exline, J.J. (2013) Religious and spiritual struggles. In *APA Handbook of Psychology, Religion, and Spirituality*. Vol. 1: Context, theory, and research (eds K.I. Pargament, J.J. Exline & J. Jones): pp. 459–76. American Psychological Association.

Exline, J.J., Park, C.L., Smyth, J.M., *et al* (2011) Anger toward God: social-cognitive predictors, prevalence, and links with adjustment to bereavement and cancer. *Journal of Personality and Social Psychology*, **100**, 129–48.

Exline, J.A., Pargament, K.I., Grubbs, J.G., *et al* (2014) The Religious and Spiritual Struggles scale: development and initial validation. *Psychology of Religion and Spirituality*, **6**, 208–22.

Fetzer Institute & National Institute on Aging Working Group (1999) *Multidimensional Measurement of Religiousness/Spirituality for Use in Health Research*. John E. Fetzer Institute.

Fontana, A. & Rosenheck, R. (2004) Trauma, change in strength of religious faith, and mental health service use among veterans treated for PTSD. *Journal of Nervous and Mental Disease*, **192**, 579–84.

Frankl, V. (1984) *Man's Search for Meaning*. Washington Square Press.

Gall, T.L. & Guirguis-Younger, M. (2013) Religious and spiritual coping: current theory and research. In *APA Handbook of Psychology, Religion, and Spirituality*. Vol. 1: Context, theory, and research (eds K.I. Pargament, J.J. Exline & J. Jones): pp. 349–64. American Psychological Association.

Geertz, C. (1966) Religion as a cultural system. In *Anthropological Approaches to the Study of Religion* (ed. M. Banton): pp. 1–46. Tavistock.

Granqvist, P. & Kirkpatrick, L.A. (2013) Religion, spirituality, and attachment. In *APA Handbook of Psychology, Religion, and Spirituality*. Vol. 1: Context, theory, and research (eds K.I. Pargament, J.J. Exline & J. Jones): pp. 139–58. American Psychological Association.

Johnson, P.E. (1959) *The Psychology of Religion*. Abingdon Press.

Karff, S.E. (2005) *Permission to Believe*. Abingdon Press.

Kirkpatrick, L.A. (2005) *Attachment, Evolution, and the Psychology of Religion*. Guilford Press.

Kirov, G., Kemp, R., Kirov, K., et al (1998) Religious faith after psychotic illness. *Psychopathology*, **31**, 234–45.

Koenig, H.G., King, D. & Carson, V.B. (2012) (eds) *Handbook of Religion and Health*, 2nd edn. Oxford University Press.

Lomax, J.W., Kripal, J.J. & Pargament, K.I. (2011) Perspectives on 'sacred moments' in psychotherapy. *American Journal of Psychiatry*, **168**, 1–7.

McConnell, K.M., Pargament, K.I., Ellison, C.G., et al (2006) Examining the links between spiritual struggles and symptoms of psychopathology in a national sample. *Journal of Clinical Psychology*, **62**, 1469–84.

McCullough, M.E., & Carter, E.C. (2013) Religion, self-control, and self-regulation: how and why are they related? In *APA Handbook of Psychology, Religion, and Spirituality*. Vol. 1: Context, theory, and research (eds K.I. Pargament, J.J. Exline & J. Jones): pp. 123–38. American Psychological Association.

Meissner, W.W. (1984) *Psychoanalysis and Religious Experience*. Yale University Press.

Mohr, S., Brandt, P.Y., Borras, L., et al (2006) Toward an integration of religiousness and spirituality into the psychosocial dimension of schizophrenia. *American Journal of Psychiatry*, **163**, 1952–9.

Mohr, S., Perroud, N., Gilleron, C., et al (2011) Spirituality and religiousness as predictive factors of outcome in schizophrenia and schizo-affective disorders. *Psychiatry Research*, **186**, 177–82.

Murray-Swank, N.A. & Waelde, L.C. (2013) Spirituality, religion, and sexual trauma: Integrating research, theory, and clinical practice. In *APA Handbook of Psychology, Religion, and Spirituality*. Vol. 2: An applied psychology of religion and spirituality (eds K.I. Pargament, A. Mahoney. & E. Shafranske): pp. 335–54. American Psychological Association.

Neeleman, J. & Lewis, G. (1994) Religious identity and comfort beliefs in three groups of psychiatric patients and a group of medical controls. *International Journal of Social Psychiatry*, **40**, 124–34.

Pargament, K.I. (2007) *Spiritually Integrated Psychotherapy: Understanding and Addressing the Sacred*. Guilford Press.

Pargament, K.I. (2011) Religion and coping: the current state of knowledge. In *Oxford Handbook of Stress, Health, and Coping* (ed. S. Folkman): pp. 269–88. Oxford University Press.

Pargament, K.I. (2013) Searching for the sacred: Toward a non-reductionistic theory of spirituality. In *APA Handbook of Psychology, Religion, and Spirituality*. Vol. 1: Context, theory, and research (eds K.I. Pargament, J.J. Exline & J. Jones): pp. 257–74. American Psychological Association.

Pargament, K.I. & Park, C.L. (1995) Merely a defense: the variety of religious means and ends. *Journal of Social Issues*, **51**, 13–32.

Pargament, K.I., Koenig, H.G., Tarakeshwar, N., et al (2004) Religious coping methods as predictors of psychological, physical, and spiritual outcomes among medically ill elderly patients: a two-year longitudinal study. *Journal of Health Psychology*, **9**, 713–30.

Pargament, K.I., Murray-Swank, N., Magyar, G., et al (2005) Spiritual struggle: a phenomenon of interest to psychology and religion. In *Judeo-Christian Perspectives on Psychology: Human Nature, Motivation, and Change* (eds W.R. Miller, H. Delaney): pp. 245–68. APA Press.

Park, C.L. (2013) Why religion? Meaning as motivation. In *APA Handbook of Psychology, Religion, and Spirituality*. Vol 1, Context, theory, and research (eds K.I. Pargament, J.J. Exline & J. Jones): pp. 157–72. American Psychological Association.

Phillips, R.E. & Stein, C.H. (2007) God's will, God's punishment, or God's limitations? Religious coping strategies reported by young adults living with serious mental illness. *Journal of Clinical Psychology*, **63**, 529–40.

Rizutto, A.M. (1979) *The Birth of the Living God: A Psychoanalytic Study*. University of Chicago Press.

Rosmarin, D.H., Bigda-Peyton, J.S., Ongur, D., *et al* (2013) Religious coping among psychotic patients: relevance to suicidality and treatment outcomes. *Psychiatric Research*, **210**, 182–7.

Smith, T.B., Bartz, J.D. & Richards, P.S. (2007) Outcomes of religious and spiritual adaptations to psychotherapy: a meta-analytic review. *Psychotherapy Research*, **17**,643–55.

Tepper, L., Rogers, S.A., Coleman, E.M., *et al* (2001) The prevalence of religious coping among persons with persistent mental illness. *Psychiatric Services*, **52**, 660–5.

Vaillant, G.E. (2002) *Aging Well*. Little Brown.

CHAPTER 6

# Stories of joy and sorrow: spirituality and affective disorder

Frederic C. Craigie, Jr

A 51-year-old government worker recounts:

> I was overwhelmed. It seemed like everywhere I turned, things were wrong… things didn't make sense. Finances were bad and I got behind on car payments and the mortgage, and the bank was calling me. My son and his wife were going through a painful divorce, and my wife seemed pretty aloof with me… I guess I was with her, too. There was a lot of pressure at work… two of the people who share the work with me went out on medical leave… they couldn't take it… and that left me holding the bag (and not holding it very well). Migraine headaches… it was pretty bad. My doctor said I was depressed, which I'm sure was true, and set me up with a psychiatrist. I saw her a couple of times. She said she could put me on medicine, but she thought that just getting going walking would be as helpful, and I did that. I don't think I can tell you anything particular that she said, but I mainly just remember that she really seemed to believe in me. She saw something in me beyond what I was going through. I distinctly remember walking one day and realizing that they could take everything away from me, but they couldn't take away my soul. I think that was the point when I really began to turn it around.

Affective disorders the literature predominantly refers to as 'depression' are extremely prevalent, with rates of current depression estimated at around 9% in the USA (Centers for Disease Control, 2010) and in Europe (Ayuso-Mateos et al, 2001). Rates of depression in people already in the healthcare system are even higher (Strosahl, 1997). Considered at a population level, these numbers are staggering. Considered at an individual level, there are, as the chapter title suggests, a great number of 'stories of sorrow' among us.

Readers of this book do not need to be reminded of the diagnostic criteria associated with affective disorders. From a narrative perspective, however, the suffering that these numbers reflect runs deeper than objective diagnostic criteria. For many people depression involves a profound loss of sense of self, of meaningful personal direction, and of a sense of 'agency' and empowerment to live their lives in faithfulness to what really matters. The suffering and the remediation of suffering (as the government worker suggests) often occur at the level of the 'soul'.

In this chapter, I shall briefly review some literature on spirituality and affective disorders, and then present a number of approaches and examples of narrative-based, spiritually informed clinical care. Given recent data about the dubious benefit of medication treatment for mild to moderate depression (Fournier *et al*, 2010), it may be that these approaches have particular relevance to patients whose disorders fall in these ranges. However, there are some data about the benefits of psychosocial treatment of even severe depression (DeRubeis *et al*, 1999) and data that the skills associated with psychosocial treatment can attenuate the possibility of relapse (Hollon *et al*, 2005), so these approaches may be relevant for psychiatrists and other clinicians as they work with patients across a wide spectrum of distress.

## Spirituality and affective disorders

There are hundreds of cross-sectional and longitudinal studies of the association of spiritual beliefs and practices with mood disorder and distress. Koenig (2012) provides a particularly helpful meta-analytic review of these associations. Examining over 3300 studies (with 600 citations) of spiritual/religious variables with various mental and physical health conditions, he found that two-thirds of studies of depression showed inverse (i.e. favourable) relationships between spiritual/religious variables and depression, and 6–7% showed unfavourable relationships. These findings parallel those of a recent meta-analytic review of spirituality and mental disorders (Bonelli & Koenig, 2013), which found 79% of studies on depression reporting inverse relationships.

Intervention trials offer richer interpretive possibilities and clinical implications. Some examples of clinical intervention studies that expressly refer to and draw upon spiritual traditions and approaches are:

- an 8-week, audiotaped spirituality home-study programme (meaning and purpose, connectedness, compassion, acceptance, love and forgiveness) (Rickhi *et al*, 2011)
- a 4-day spiritual retreat for depression in patients with acute coronary syndrome (meditation, guided imagery, journaling, drawing, and nature activities and imagery) (Warber *et al*, 2011)
- eight-session spiritually integrated psychotherapy ('emotional-spiritual methods with religious content' with components of control, meaning-finding, identity and communication) (Ebrahimi *et al*, 2013)
- group instruction with individual follow-up of choosing and using spiritual mantra derived from world spiritual traditions (Bormann *et al*, 2006)
- individual direct-contact prayer, with 6 weekly 1 h sessions (Boelens *et al*, 2012).

In addition, there are a number of clinical intervention models that refer variously (or not at all) to 'spirituality' but are informed by spiritual traditions and approaches. These include:

- mindfulness-based approaches (Würtzen *et al*, 2013)
- acceptance and commitment therapy (Karlin *et al*, 2013)
- life review (Ando *et al*, 2008)
- cognitive–behavioural therapy (Williams *et al*, 2013)
- compassion-focused therapy (Heriot-Maitland *et al*, 2014)
- mindful self-compassion (Neff & Germer, 2013).

# Narrative in spiritual care

What we call 'spirituality' is a rich and multi-dimensional human experience. There are multiple pathways for understanding spirituality and for drawing on spiritual practices and perspectives in clinical care. The common element that weaves together these pathways is that they invite people to develop new stories of their lives.

> 'I was seriously abused emotionally and sexually [when I was] growing up. I've been working on making peace with my history for a long time... psychotherapy, my church relationships, my writing, my poetry, my second husband, who is incredibly supportive... a lot of things have helped along the way. The bottom line is that I used to see myself as "damaged goods", and now I'm able to see myself as having something to offer to the world. I'll always have my history, but that's not the definition of who I am any more. I feel really blessed and full.'

Spirituality invites new and deeply important narratives about who people are and how they live their lives. As new narratives unfold, people who are emotionally adrift develop stories of purpose and direction. People with chronic and serious illnesses develop stories of resilience. People whose attention and hearts are scattered develop stories of mindfulness and presence. People who are disconnected develop stories of connectedness. People who are bitter and vengeful develop new stories of forgiveness. People who are besieged by multiple life challenges remember what is ultimately important. And sometimes, people with stories of sorrow come to find new narratives of hope and joy.

I want to explore two principal conversations to help people in developing these new narratives, drawing both on empirical research and on many years of dialogue about spiritual care. As a preface, however, let me begin with two items about the context.

## *Intention and presence*

First, as in exploring approaches to supporting people in developing new narratives, I want to affirm the foundational importance of our own groundedness, healing intention and compassionate presence. We engage techniques but we are not technicians.

A recent patient visited a complementary care provider and commented:

> 'The acupuncture was great, but what was most remarkable was how clearly he really cared about me and who I am. I look at people's eyes... I could see it in his eyes that I was more than a "patient". I went away just feeling... loved.'

Sometimes, indeed, our healing intention and compassionate presence may be the most powerful gift that we give our patients as they explore new narratives – as with the government worker, who did not remember much of what the psychiatrist said, but recalled that 'she really seemed to believe in me. She saw something in me beyond what I was going through'. At other times, our intention and presence lay the groundwork for collaborative, partnership relationships.

## *The vital and sacred*

Second, how we think about spirituality informs how we work with spirituality in clinical care. There is a fine and rich definition of spirituality from the Royal College of Psychiatrists earlier in this volume (p. 5). My favourite succinct definition of spirituality, one that often anchors the conversation for me about spirituality in clinical care, comes from former US Surgeon General C. Everett Koop, MD:

> 'The vital center of a person; that which is held sacred.' (Koop, 1994)

The ideas of vitality (whose Latin word root *vita* means 'life') and sacredness point to a depth of human values and experience that may direct and energize people's journeys away from emotional darkness and towards healing. Spiritual care consists of helping people to understand and cultivate 'vital and sacred' values and qualities in their lives (Craigie, 2010):

> 'Helping people to connect with the things that really matter to them' (p. 88).

In the 2011 documentary film *Fambul Tok* ('Family talk'), an emotionally destitute perpetrator of violence is touched by an invitation to forgiveness and reconciliation by his community in Sierra Leone and reflects:

> 'I need to get my life… I haven't been living my life… I've just been doing things.'

Particularly with mood disorders, people often gravitate to a position of 'doing things' (or not) but not 'living life'. The heartfelt comment that this man makes about 'living life' captures well the spiritual quest to define and give expression to 'what really matters' or to 'principles that are at the core of their being', or to personal values and qualities that are 'vital and sacred'.

## Two core processes in spiritual care with mood disorders: purpose and transcendence

There are two important, recurring and complementary conversations that frame how I think about spiritually informed narrative work with people with mood disorders. They are conversations about 'purpose' and 'transcendence'.

'Purpose' means living life in faithfulness to deeply important personal values. A psychologist describes:

'A woman came in to talk about mood issues. I was struck looking at her health record at what a painful history she had. She had three or four suicide attempts and had been hospitalized seven times. She had accumulated a remarkable collection of psychiatric diagnoses. I did notice, though, that she had neither a suicide attempt nor an in-patient mental health hospital admission in the past 3 years. I'm always interested in how people make positive changes in their lives, and I asked her what she thought was going on. She said that her parents had largely been absent in her life and she was raised by retirement-aged neighbours, for whom she had great fondness. Three years ago, the woman passed away, leaving the man emotionally adrift. She had taken it upon herself to care for him, living with him for a while and then seeing him and supporting him regularly. She said she thought that this caring relationship was what helped her to let go of her struggle with depression and move forward in her own life. Ever interested in how people make changes, I asked her how she would put into words why this had been important. She said "It gave me a reason for living, a purpose for being on this planet".'

'Transcendence' (literally, 'moving across or rising above some difficulty or obstacle') means being able to 'let go' or 'make peace' with experiences that are outside of our control. These can be external experiences (such as the behaviour of other people and features of the physical environment) and internal experiences (such as unbidden and unwelcome thoughts, feelings, images and physical sensations).

'As he wrestled with mood issues, a patient told the story of dealing with his younger brother's death. They had been snowmobiling together, on a day that turned grey with heavy snow and limited visibility. The brother got out ahead and when my patient caught up to him, he found his snowmobile upturned in the woods to the side of the trail. The brother lay nearby, having apparently been killed instantly by running into a tree. My patient, of course, was devastated. In weeks following the incident, he said that he was plagued by terrifying images of the accident scene and his brother's stunned expression, and by thoughts that if he had only been a more responsible older brother and had them both head back home slowly, this would not have happened. He found himself depressed and increasingly isolated from his normal life. Over time, though, he said he had realized that these images and thoughts had been taking over his life, and he did not want to give that power to them. He wished to be "responsible" for his parents and for his brother's grown children. He concluded "I came to understand that I can't control my thoughts and feelings, and I learned to let them come, let them do their thing, but focus for myself on what I need to be doing".'

Purpose and transcendence are complementary elements of change and healing. Purpose – moving forward in faithfulness to vital personal values – often requires the ability to let go or make peace with unchangeable experiences. The snowmobiling brother would have been less well able to do what he needed to do and be responsible for his remaining family if he had not reached some accommodation with his brother's death and with the images and thoughts that it prompted. Transcendence – letting go of unchangeable outer and inner experiences – is often energized by some vital purpose. The woman who cared for her neighbour would have been less able to let go of her own struggle with depression if she had not had the vital and sacred purpose of extending love and care to this man to whom she felt so devoted.

## Cultivating purpose

How might we support patients in identifying and cultivating purpose in narrative-oriented spiritual care conversations in the setting of mood disorders? Let us look at some ideas and approaches.

### Conversational approaches to purpose

A 'mantra' that I frequently suggest to our residents comes from organizational consultant Margaret Wheatley (2009):

> 'Real change begins with the simple act of people talking about what they care about' (p. 22)

Inviting people to talk about the things they care about provides direction and, more importantly, brings 'energy' into the room. This invitation takes countless forms:

- What do you really care about?
- What matters to you?
- What is sacred for you?
- What is your life 'about'?
- What do you hope the legacy of your life would be?
- What keeps you going?
- What is there about your life that you take pride in?
- When do you feel really 'alive'?
- What motivates you to want to make this change?
- How would you put into words... (why this matters to you, what kind of person you'd like to be, how you hope you'd be handling this, etc.)?

See this example conversation between a patient and clinician:

CLINICIAN: So this really has been a hard time for you, and I can see the suffering and how stalled out you have felt. How would you put into words what you want at this point... what should we be working on together?

PATIENT: I just want to be happy... again.

CLINICIAN: 'Happy, again'... OK, can you say more about what 'happy' means to you?

PATIENT: I'm so down, I can't...

CLINICIAN: OK... think of a time that was a pretty good time for you, a time when you had more of a sense of happiness.

PATIENT: I was pretty happy when I owned my business.

CLINICIAN: What was that – can you give me a picture of that?

PATIENT: It was a used book store. I would sit at the front, these big piles of books all around me... back then, you could smoke indoors and I had a pipe going most of the time. People would come in and I would have these conversations about books and authors and... life, I guess.

CLINICIAN: That was a good time for you.
PATIENT: Yea, it was.
CLINICIAN: How would you put into words why that mattered to you?
PATIENT: I don't know... the books, the people...
CLINICIAN: OK, the books, the people... what is it about you that made books and people important to you?
PATIENT: You know, when I think about it, it was like I created almost a sacred place... being there, just relating to ideas and to people with ideas.

The clinician is inviting the patient to give voice to what really matters to him. In conversational approaches to purpose, this invitation may take forms both of asking the kinds of questions that are bulleted above, and of picking up on and inviting elaboration of patients' constructs and language that may potentially begin to form new narratives. This conversation might proceed by establishing the fact that 'relating to ideas' is a core value for this person, and exploring how this value could offer direction and energy in the journey of healing. The clinician might also pick up on the patient's use of the word 'sacred' and explore what this means to the patient and how this word may open the conversation to particular spiritual beliefs and practices.

In general, the process of inviting elaboration of what people say that may help to form new narratives may focus on several elements:

- *Vision.* Most patients who have been in the system for some time are expert at telling their stories of suffering. What, in contrast, are they saying about what they want? Where do they hope to be going? How might they hope their lives would be different?
- *Values.* What are they saying about what matters to them (e.g. 'relating to ideas', as in the example patient–clinician exchange above)?
- *Agency.* In some countries, there are a number of forces (direct-to-consumer advertising among them) that present a model of depression in which patients are passive recipients of care that comes from outside them. What are patients saying about their own abilities to make changes that move them towards new narratives?
- *Competence.* One of my hallowed rules for our residents is 'Catch patients in the act of being competent'. Generally, we know the story of incapacity and incompetence. What, in contrast, are patients saying about how they have accomplished something meaningful to them, and how did they do this?
- *Language.* Finally, what language and metaphors are patients using that may point the way to new narratives? I recently asked a young man about his tattoos and he said that they related to his 'spirituality'. How would he describe what his 'spirituality' means to him? He said that at his best, he thinks of himself as 'a Jedi'. Both of these words, 'spirituality' and 'Jedi' come from the patient. He has ownership of these words and they potentially offer rich and personally meaningful possibilities of new directions.

As we think about spiritual care, I believe the issue of language warrants special emphasis. My practice is that I rarely introduce spiritual language in questions and conversations. I am vigilant, however, in looking for words that patients use that may signify some spiritual beliefs or practices, and I pick up on these words when I hear them. Some questions about coping and depth of experience, moreover, often elicit spiritual language and world views:

- What keeps you going?
- Where do you turn to make sense of things like this?
- Where do you turn to find comfort in hard times like these?

See this next example: .

CLINICIAN: I can see your struggle with the suicidal thoughts. Let me ask you, what keeps you going?

PATIENT: My wife and my faith.

CLINICIAN: Your wife…?

PATIENT: Yes, it would just devastate her… her world would end.

CLINICIAN: Your love for her really keeps you going. And your 'faith'?

PATIENT: Well, I'm not very religious but I believe in God, and God has sometimes got me through some hard times.

CLINICIAN: When you say that God has helped you through hard times, say more…

In this example, the words 'faith' and 'God' are introduced by the patient. The patient has 'ownership' of this language. Exploring what these words mean, therefore, and exploring the world views that they signify, becomes both clinically viable and ethically unassailable.

## Exercises in defining purpose

There are countless self-reflective exercises that can help people to begin to develop 'vital' and 'sacred' aspects of their lives. Here are some examples.

- *Three adjectives.* 'Write three words or short phrases that would capture what it is that you most want to be like as a person'. A patient responded, 'Honest, caring… making a difference in the world, and being the kind of person my children can be proud of'.
- *Going away celebration.* 'If you were going to relocate to a far-away community and there was a gathering in your honour, what would you hope people might say about you in tribute?'
- *Someone who loves you.* 'What would I hear about you if I were talking with someone who knows you well and loves you, someone who is able to see the best in you?'
- *You at your best.* 'Tell a story about a day-to-day event. This might be something that other people are not even aware of, but that shows something about you at your best.' My experience is that people very frequently describe small acts of generosity or kindness.
- *All I have to do.* 'Fill in the blank: All I have to do is _____'. This exercise originated in comments from a physician as she completed

the integrative medicine fellowship where I teach. Reflecting on what she had learned about integrative medicine and doctoring during the 2-year fellowship, she said she would always be devoted and professionally accountable in her work, but that she had realised that 'Ultimately, all I have to do is love'.

## Moving forward with purpose

Change may be planned in conversations with professionals, but change happens in the world. Developing action steps towards realizing purpose consists of bringing together what I call 'patient wisdom' and 'clinician wisdom'.

- 'Patient wisdom' means drawing upon patients' own life experiences and thoughts about moving forward.

   > CLINICIAN 1: 'Caring and making a difference', OK. When has there been a time in your life when you've felt like you were doing this? Let's look at this and think about how it might apply to where you are now.

   > CLINICIAN 2: So you're saying that 'faithfulness to the Lord' has mattered so deeply to you. Let's build on that. If you were 20% more 'faithful to the Lord' in the next couple of weeks, what would that look like?

- 'Clinician wisdom' about moving forward means proposing our own ideas about directions patients might pursue to more fully realize spiritual values. Clinician wisdom takes three forms:
   a. This is what the data say: 'When you look at the research about what is called "behavioural activation", what you see is...'
   b. This is what my patients have said: 'I had a patient a couple of weeks ago who was really interested in being able to be more mindful and present. What he said he discovered was...'
   c. This has been my personal experience: 'I think what you are wrestling with about creativity, how you take it from here, is really important. Let me toss out a couple of ideas that I have seen in myself about song-writing...'

## *Transcendence*

Along with purpose, the other element of new narratives with mood disorders is transcendence. The new narrative is one of living in faithfulness to sacred values, and it is also one of letting go or making peace with unchangeable, uninvited, unpleasant experiences. The abused woman I quoted earlier (p. 69) said that she had come to recognize that she would 'always have my history,' but that 'that's not the definition of who I am'. She had come to an accommodation with her painful history; it was still 'there', but no longer had power over her life.

People have all manner of uninvited and often unchangeable life experiences and suffering that pose emotional barriers to living fully and well, and which they are challenged to transcend or 'release'. These include 'external' challenges such as past trauma or critical or demeaning family members, and 'internal' challenges such as intrusive images, pain, thoughts of inadequacy and self-blame, and feelings of anxiety, vengefulness or hopelessness. There are several approaches to transcendence that derive from spiritual traditions and from psychological practice and we will look at them in detail now.

### Letting go

Letting go does not have any foundation in empirical research, but I mention it because it can be so much a part of the common parlance. The idea of letting go is widely understood, generally acceptable and non-threatening to consider. It can provide a viable linguistic anchor for conversations about transcending uninvited and unchangeable life experiences and suffering. I frequently find the question 'What do you think you'll have to let go of in order to move forward as you want?' to be a helpful conversation starter.

### Acceptance/willingness

These words derive especially from the empirical literature about acceptance and commitment therapy. 'Acceptance' means developing the ability to tolerate unwelcome and unpleasant experiences ('outer' and 'inner') without avoidance. 'Willingness' means intentionally facing circumstances that are likely to prompt unpleasant experiences, in the interest of having a fuller life:

> When I was most depressed, it was really hard for me even to go out the door. I guess I felt so down on myself that I felt like people were watching me and they'd see that I was stupid and ugly. I couldn't look people in the eye. It was a lot easier just to stay home. I realized eventually that the more preoccupied I got with what people would think of me and the more I kept safe in my home, [the more] I was just 'feeding the wolf'. I decided that even if I had these voices that told me I was a loser, and even if I was going to feel so anxious that I couldn't put two words together, I wasn't going to feed the wolf any more. The more I got out, it felt like I was meeting myself again for the first time in a long time.

### Mindfulness/being present

While the word 'mindfulness' may signify particular meditative practices ('mindfulness meditation', 'loving-kindness meditation'), mindfulness is foremost a way of relating to the world. Three elements of mindfulness are:

- paying attention, being aware
- in the present moment
- without judgement.

When people are distressed and depressed, their attention, focus and heart are almost always located in the past or the future. Mindfulness means gently drawing your attention and heart back to the present moment – which really is all there is anyway. How, you might ask, does your patient wish to be living their life in this one sacred, irreplaceable moment? Current psychological/spiritual literature has abundant empirical work and commentary on mindfulness and being present (Khoury *et al*, 2013).

### Non-attachment

The idea of non-attachment has its origins in Eastern and Buddhist philosophy. We learn to live with the paradox that we care and we do not care. I care deeply about the patients I work with and hold the great hope that I may in some way enrich their lives. But the other half of the paradox is that I do not care. If a person who misuses substances goes back to using, or a person with depression resolutely stays at home watching television, I can care deeply about them, but I cannot and do not care that they have made those choices about their own, autonomous lives. I care about the outcome, but I am not attached to the outcome. Similarly, a colleague commented that we have to be 'passionate and dispassionate'. For our patients, the idea of non-attachment is just the same as it is for us.

### Serenity

In America, serenity is most often associated with the 'serenity prayer', which was fashioned from 18th-century roots by Protestant theologian Reinhold Niebuhr and is frequently quoted in the 12-step movement. Most frequently cited is the first stanza:

> 'God, grant me the serenity to accept things I cannot change,
> The courage to change the things I can,
> And the wisdom to know the difference.'

I find that serenity is widely understood in this form, and for many people provides an accessible and meaningful way to approach the ideas we have been considering about transcendence and purpose.

### Gratitude/gratefulness

The practice of gratitude or gratefulness reflects ancient spiritual wisdom. In the Judaic tradition, the sacred texts, the Psalms for example, are rich with expressions of thanksgiving to God. In the Islamic tradition, the daily practice of *Salat* (prayer) focuses the worshipper in a relationship of adoration and gratitude to God. In the Christian tradition, Paul of Tarsus instructs the church in Thessalonica to be 'thankful in all circumstances, for this is God's will for you'.

In all of these traditions, gratitude does not mean situation-specific thankfulness, as you would say 'thanks' when someone offers you a cup of tea. It is a spiritual practice and an attitude towards daily living. The spiritual underpinning of this practice is that an attitude of gratefulness helps people to be open to the creative and healing movement of God even in challenging circumstances.

Modern research points to a variety of emotional and health benefits of gratefulness, which is usually operationalized as daily or weekly gratitude journals (Emmons & Stern, 2013). I find that gratitude journals help people not only to 'count their blessings', but to see meaningful possibilities inherent in challenging circumstances. The benefit in terms of transcendence is that gratitude may help people to move away from the reflexive, judgemental categorization of daily events as 'good' or 'bad'.

**Forgiveness**

Like gratitude, forgiveness has ancient spiritual roots. Also like gratitude, there is a modern empirical research base that attests to a variety of emotional and health benefits of extending forgiveness (Wade *et al*, 2014). This is not surprising. As much as anything else, people I see with mood disorders are held captive by narratives of woundedness at the hands of other people. Forgiveness frees people from this captivity and allows them to live purposefully. As I explore forgiveness with patients, I see five recurring elements.

1. Forgiveness is unilateral. It releases those who have injured from the prospect of retribution, thereby releasing the shackles that hold victims emotionally and spiritually to woundedness, and freeing them to invest energy in meaningful living. Reconciliation is bilateral when those who have injured choose to join in the process of acknowledging the reality of the injury and pursuing a restoration of relationship.
2. Forgiveness must be grounded in acknowledgement of feelings associated with mistreatment and injuries.
3. Forgiveness is a process of working through mistreatment; it is not a snap or shallow decision.
4. Forgiveness typically involves coming to see those who have injured in a new light, with intellectual understanding and often with empathy.
5. Forgiveness is paradoxical; by extending forgiveness to other people, we promote our own healing.

Particularly with narrative approaches, I suggest that the idea of forgiveness is often best approached by storytelling:

> 'I remember a patient who had been raised largely by her mum after her parents divorced. She had been verbally abused for a long time by an alcoholic father who had been removed from the home when he abused her physically. She hadn't seen him in years and always found herself bitter and vengeful when she thought of him. She had to go to Boston, were he lives, and when she was driving down, she heard a voice saying "You can't go on like this". She added that she didn't really hear a voice but she had a strong urge to go see him. She drove in the driveway and he came out the door and she said she just hugged him and said "I love you". He was stunned. She took him out to lunch and they talked. She said it wasn't an earth-shaking conversation and she's not sure where their relationship might go from here, but she said "Mainly I felt like a great weight had been lifted off my shoulders. I knew at that point, it was about me. I had to forgive him... even if he doesn't deserve it... because my bitterness was going to eat me like a cancer. I feel like I've reclaimed that part of my life".'

Self-forgiveness, I might add, often holds similar importance and follows similar paths to forgiveness of others.

## Staying connected

If we think of spiritual care as supporting 'connections with things that matter' (whether this might mean personal qualities, commitments to relationships or other meaningful values), then the challenge for our patients is both to develop and to maintain these connections. Therefore, encouraging ongoing self-reflective practices can be a vital element of spiritual care. Examples include:

- Daily centring practices: meditative practices, mindful walking (in expressly spiritual spaces such as labyrinths (Curry, 2000) or just in the course of daily movement), reading of sacred texts, contemplation or prayer.
- Affirmations: the 12-step tradition has a rich collection of affirmations (the word they use is 'aphorisms') – 'One day at a time', 'Let go and let God', 'First things first'. How might your patient capture in a few words the essence of what they wish they remain focused on along their journey of healing?
- Journaling: Regular, written self-reflection.
- Sustained movement: I have heard from many people (and this has been my experience as well) that sustained, private, non-interactive movement like jogging, swimming or cycling can foster a state of mindfulness and openness to intuition and insights. In many of the comments that I hear, this openness brings with it a fresher awareness of what matters.
- Retreats: retreats provide an additional approach/methodology for staying connected with what matters (the word 'retreat' originates in the 1400s, meaning 'to draw in, draw back, fall back from battle'). The experience of retreating can be meaningful and the venues to which one retreats are often sacred or spiritually uplifting places.
- Community: interpersonal connections can help us all to focus on shared values and to be accountable to upholding them. Religious or spiritual communities, fraternal and civic organizations, collaborative teams and good friendships can all support our patients' understanding and experience of purpose and transcendence.

## Conclusions

We have been looking at clinical approaches that can support patients in developing new narratives of their lives, anchored in what is deeply meaningful and 'vital and sacred' for them. The conversations we have with people in spiritually informed care rest on a foundation of healing intention and compassionate presence, and explore the complementary ideas of 'purpose' and 'transcendence' in a collaborative, patient-centred way.

# References

Ando, M., Morita, T., Okamoto, T., et al (2008) One-week short term life review can improve spiritual well-being of terminally ill cancer patients. *Psycho-Oncology*, **17**, 885–90.

Ayuso-Mateos, J.L., Vazquez-Barquero, J.L., Dowrick, C., et al (2001) Depressive disorders in Europe: prevalence figures from the ODIN study. *British Journal of Psychiatry*, **179**, 308–16.

Boelens, P.A., Reeves, R.R., Replogle, W.H., et al (2012) The effect of prayer on depression and anxiety: maintenance of positive influence one year after prayer intervention. *International Journal of Psychiatry in Medicine*, **43**, 85–98.

Bonelli, R.M. & Koenig, H.G. (2013) Mental disorders, religion and spirituality 1990 to 2010: a systematic evidence-based review. *Journal of Religion and Health*, **52**, 657–73.

Bormann, J.E., Gifford, A.L. Shively, M., et al (2006) Effects of spiritual mantram repetition on HIV outcomes: a randomized controlled trial. *Journal of Behavioral Medicine*, **29**, 359–76.

Centers for Disease Control (2010) Current depression among adults – United States, 2006 and 2008. *Morbidity and Mortality Weekly Report*, **59**, 1229–35.

Craigie, F.C. (2010) *Positive Spirituality in Health Care: Nine Practical Approaches to Pursuing Wholeness for Clinicians, Patients, and Health Care Organizations*. Mill City Press.

Curry, H. (2000) *The Way of the Labyrinth: A Powerful Meditation for Everyday Life*. Penguin Compass.

DeRubeis, R.J., Gelfand, L.A., Tang, T.Z., et al (1999) Medications versus cognitive behavior therapy for severely depressed outpatients: mega-analysis of four randomized comparisons. *American Journal of Psychiatry*, **156**, 1007–13.

Ebrahimi, A., Neshatdoost, H.T., Mousavi, S.G., et al (2013) Controlled randomized clinical trial of spirituality integrated psychotherapy, cognitive-behavioral therapy and medication intervention on depressive symptoms and dysfunctional attitudes in patients with dysthymic disorder. *Advanced Biomedical Research*, **2**, 53.

Emmons, R.A. & Stern, R. (2013) Gratitude as a psychotherapeutic intervention. *Journal of Clinical Psychology*, **69**, 846–55.

Fournier, J.C., DeRubeis, R.J., Hollon, S.D., et al (2010) Antidepressant drug effects and depression severity: a patient-level meta-analysis. *JAMA*, **303**, 47–53.

Heriot-Maitland, C., Vidal, J.B., Ball, S., et al (2014) A compassionate-focused therapy group approach for acute inpatients: feasibility, initial pilot outcome data, and recommendations. *British Journal of Clinical Psychology*, **53**, 78–94.

Hollon, S.D., DeRubeis, R.J., Shelton, R.C., et al (2005) Prevention of relapse following cognitive therapy vs medications in moderate to severe depression. *Archives of General Psychiatry*, **62**, 417–22.

Karlin, B.E., Walser, R.D., Yesavage, J., et al (2013) Effectiveness of acceptance and commitment therapy for depression: comparison among older and younger veterans. *Aging Mental Health*, **17**, 555–63.

Khoury, B., Lecomte, T., Fortin, G., et al (2013) Mindfulness-based therapy: a comprehensive meta-analysis. *Clinical Psychology Review*, **33**, 763–71.

Koenig, H.G. (2012) Religion, spirituality, and health: the research and clinical implications. *ISRN Psychiatry*, 16 December, doi: 10.5402/2012/278730. [Epub.]

Koop, C.E. (1994) Spirituality and Health Promotion: Clinical Care, Community Responsibility and Public Policy. Keynote presentation at the 8th Annual Thomas Nevola, MD Symposium on Spirituality and Health, Augusta, Maine.

Neff, K.D. & Germer, C.K. (2013) A pilot study and randomized controlled trial of the mindful self-compassion program. *Journal of Clinical Psychology*, **69**, 28–44.

Rickhi, B., Moritz, S., Reesal, R., et al (2011) A spirituality teaching program for depression: a randomized controlled trial. *International Journal of Psychiatry in Medicine*, **42**, 315–29.

Strosahl, K. (1997) Building primary care behavioral health systems that work: a compass and a horizon. In *Behavioral Health in Primary Care* (eds N. Cummings, J. Cummings, J. Johnson): pp. 37–58. Psychosocial Press.

Wade, N.G., Hoyt, W.T., Kidwell, J.E., *et al* (2014) Efficacy of psychotherapeutic interventions to promote forgiveness: a meta-analysis. *Journal of Clinical and Consulting Psychology*, **82**, 154–70.

Warber, S.L., Ingerman, S., Moura, V.L., *et al* (2011) Healing the heart: a randomized pilot study of a spiritual retreat for depression in acute coronary syndrome patients. *Explore (NY)*, **7**, 222–33.

Wheatley, M.J. (2009) *Turning to One Another: Simple Conversations to Restore Hope to the Future*. Berrett-Koehler.

Williams, C., Wilson, P., Morrison, J., *et al* (2013) Guided self-help behavioural therapy for depression in primary care: a randomized controlled trial. *PLoS ONE*, **8**, e52735.

Würtzen, H., Dalton, S.O., Elsass, P., *et al* (2013) Mindfulness significantly reduces self-reported levels of anxiety and depression: results of a randomized controlled trial among 336 Danish women treated for stage I-III breast cancer. *European Journal of Cancer*, **49**, 1365–73.

CHAPTER 7

# Stories of fear: spirituality and anxiety disorders

Chris Williams

Personal faith and a spiritual perspective are important to many people, who can describe a sense of hope, meaning and purpose as a result of their beliefs. As well as providing guidance in everyday life, their faith may provide encouragement and support during difficult times such as illness. A pattern can be given to the day or week through meditation or prayer, readings from a holy book, or attendance at communal worship or groups. The person may adhere to the tenets of one or other of the world's religions, or their spirituality can more reflect their personal views.

For people who have a personal faith, or for whom a spiritual outlook is important, mental health problems can affect the content of their spiritual experiences. Likewise, a person's spiritual beliefs can affect how they experience mental health difficulties. Personal beliefs can be a positive and helpful resource, but sometimes aspects of faith can become unhelpfully drawn into the difficulties faced during times of distress.

## Narrative as an approach

Mental health difficulties are commonly associated with stigma and an avoidance of discussing problems with practitioners, family and friends (Rose *et al*, 2007). This can prevent individuals benefiting from being able to share their story with a trusted other. Whether shared with others or held privately, individuals have an internal narrative that aims to make sense of their experiences. However, since many people know little about mental and physical health problems, that narrative may contain significant errors and misunderstandings (Fagerlin, 2010). A helpful clinical approach is one that both supports an accurate and adaptive narrative that accurately identifies problems, and provides explanations as to why the person feels as they do, what they can do about it and how they might expect things to progress (Hagger & Orbell, 2003).

This chapter describes how cognitive–behavioural therapy (CBT) can be used to make sense of some very different personal responses to a mental health crisis. In matters of faith there is often a tension between belief and behaviour. Since CBT focuses similarly on thoughts and actions, it can be used sympathetically and helpfully with those who hold spiritual beliefs, providing a useful framework for understanding and integrating a spiritual perspective into treatment and thus facilitating a whole-person intervention (Beck, 1991).

## Cognitive–behavioural therapy: incorporating faith aspects into anxiety support

CBT is widely recommended in treatment guidelines, such as those from the National Institute for Health and Care Excellence (NICE, 2011), as an intervention for anxiety. From the CBT perspective, anxiety arises when the threat or danger being faced is overplayed and builds up in a person's mind. At the same time the individual underplays their capacity to cope with the problem. The result is to become overly aware of possible threats, which the person then tries to escape and avoid. This is described as the anxiety balance (Fig. 7.1).

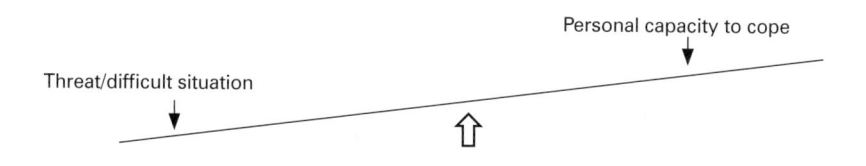

**Fig. 7.1** The anxiety balance. Source: WIlliams, 2010.

In a situation with no anxiety, the person feels in balance – they know they can cope with their problems. In contrast, in times of anxiety the balance is upset, with an unhelpful focus on problems and difficulties that are experienced as overwhelming, and the person believes they cannot cope. The result is increasing distress and altered behaviour. In this narrative, balance can be restored, first by enhancing the capacity to cope (rebalancing the right-hand side of the balance on the diagram) and/or secondly by tackling either the reality of the threat/difficult situation by using problem-solving approaches and/or thirdly by changing the perception of threat by altering the meaning of the event. The second and third methods influence the left side of the balance.

CBT formulations also encourage the person to consider what supportive relationships, as well as unsupportive relationships, they have around them. These may include a focus on re-engaging with others, building a sense of closeness in relationships, and making choices to relate to others in helpful rather than unhelpful ways.

It is in these three key domains of beliefs (including long-term rules, core beliefs and values that guide self-judgement), behaviour (what helpful and unhelpful activities are occurring) and external relationships (with people, and with God/fellow believers) that the CBT narrative is broadened to incorporate spiritual beliefs while providing a powerful alternative explanation of the experience of anxiety (Williams *et al*, 2002). These topics will be presented in three narratives.

## Farah's story

Farah is 18 years old and a Muslim, and her family originally came from Bangladesh. She went to a local private school and has been taught by her parents to dress conservatively, avoiding clothes that would reveal her shape, and to adhere to the five pillars of Islam. She sees herself as being a committed believer and follower of the Prophet and his teachings. Since adolescence she has always worn a headscarf. She has also been taught never to be alone with a boy, and that revealing her hair is something only to be done within the privacy of home or with a future husband.

To date, Farah has had only one boyfriend, also Muslim. Their friendship was largely platonic, but with occasional kisses which she enjoyed. He was a friend at school, and she could never bring him home or even tell her parents about him.

Farah is now 4 months into the first term at university. This is her first time away from home for any length of time and she lives in a shared student flat with four other girls. She categorises them by their faith – one is Muslim but from another tradition to her own, one is Christian, while the other two don't appear to follow any particular faith. As the months pass, she notices that the other girls start to have relationships and wider friendships with male students. She wants this too but feels anxious about what the right behaviour is. She gets on well with one of the male students on her degree course, Ansar. He shares Farah's beliefs but lives his faith differently. He likes to go to parties, and although he avoids alcohol, he clearly has a more open view about how men and women should relate when together. Farah finds she is attracted to him but is anxious about any physical relationship with him. She has avoided going back to Ansar's flat, since she is concerned what her parents might say if they discovered she was alone with him – even if just for a coffee.

Nevertheless, one evening she is invited to his flat and they watch a DVD together. Ansar gives her a hug which she enjoys, but then he suggests she removes her headscarf so they can hug and kiss more closely. She immediately panics, thinking 'I can't do this. What will my parents say? It's wrong'. She feels scared and breaks off, tells Ansar she feels sick and rushes out of the door. When she gets back to her flat she locks herself in her room, beating herself up mentally. She starts going over in her mind the various teachings about headscarfs she has heard over the years. Her previous imam taught that the head scarf must always be worn, whereas the Islamic workers at the university chaplaincy say that the choice is a cultural one rather than a fundamental aspect of her faith. Ansar then texts her saying he's not sure if he upset her and asks if they can meet. She deletes the text message and the next day avoids eye contact with him. She starts thinking she should just leave the course and return home.

From a CBT perspective, Farah shows key anxiety behaviours: avoidance, and rushing away from anxiety-provoking situations. She is mind-reading what others will think of her and jumping to the worst conclusions – that the only thing is to leave university completely. She doesn't want to let her faith or her parents down, yet going over the same thoughts again and again only adds to her distress. This may look like problem-solving, but actually it paralyses her. She feels in a crisis of identity, trying to work out which beliefs are fundamental to her faith and which family or societal traditions she can choose to ignore. Her distress leads to self-blame and a pattern of relating to Ansar that will probably cause him to be hurt and angry with her.

Farah's personal narrative is informed by the rules and beliefs she has learned growing up, including the beliefs of her faith group. In this case, other Muslims can be a useful source of discussion in helping Farah work out why she believes things as she does. The Islamic society worker based at the chaplaincy draws on a variety of sources to help Farah think through for herself how her beliefs, behaviour and relationships with others can be informed by her strong personal faith. She helps Farah realise that people can be true Muslims, having a devout faith and strong personal morality, and yet make different decisions about clothing and how to relate to others of the opposite gender.

This approach has much in common with CBT, resulting in Farah being able to work out what she wishes to do, talking it through with Ansar and staying on her course.

## Issues raised by Farah's story: spirituality, beliefs, behaviour

Where a personal faith and spiritual values are important to a person, the beliefs, behaviours and relationships that flow from these thoughts inform their understanding of life. This might include reminding themselves of additional resources, such as:

- The teachings, promises and alternative viewpoint offered by their faith. They may find it encouraging to study a holy book (reflecting on texts emphasising hope, stories of faithful people in the past who have faced adversity, parables and other words of wisdom, and stories of hope, reconciliation, rescue, forgiveness and God's love). The person's faith might help them take a different perspective on their suffering; that they are not alone, that God could work for the good in difficult situations, and that they have hope for the future, no matter how difficult things seem today. A spiritual perspective might therefore draw attention to the opportunities for personal growth and learning through a testing of faith. It might emphasise the personal benefits of difficulties and challenges in producing faithfulness, endurance and leaning on God or benefits such as the hope and solace provided by their faith.
- Receiving support through their faith community (including practical help, encouragement, fellowship and the promise of prayer). Feeling

loved, supported and listened to can be an important source of encouragement and hope. In Farah's case, being able to speak to someone who shares her faith helped her feel listened to, and the fact that her fears were respected and not condemned felt incredibly helpful. Visits by imams, rabbis, ministers/priests and others can reinforce this sense of being part of a wider caring community.

- The practice and application of a person's faith, through personal prayer, meditation and reflection. For someone for whom a spiritual approach to life is seen as important, personal responses might include the use of meditational strategies, mindfulness, relaxation and the potential to include prayer and study, as well as practical, problem-oriented approaches. For Farah, her practice of the five pillars of her faith can provide her with a sense of a daily pattern and time of reflection or encouragement, and the possibility of a sense of connection to, and the experience of the goodness of, God.

## Daniel's story

Daniel is 45 years old. His family background is one of Orthodox Judaism and he has always been determined to follow the ways of his forefathers. He married Sara, and they have had two children. Over recent times, Daniel and his wife had been arguing more than usual, which ended in Sara leaving him following an affair she had with a work colleague. Daniel blames himself for this, since he feels he had neglected her and the children because of the amount of work he does in his job as a teacher at the local secondary school.

Daniel has been brought up always to do his best and work hard. These beliefs colour all aspects of his life. He took his marriage vows seriously, and believes that he and Sara should have been able to work through their differences. Daniel was devastated when she left. He now feels a failure as a husband and father, and a failure before God. He thinks he should have done better, and starts to doubt himself and his decisions.

Daniel had some difficulties with obsessionality as a child, when he was very slow in writing and colouring in pictures. Later, those same traits led him to spend too much time at work instead of with his family. Obsessional–compulsive symptoms included repeatedly checking window locks and, more recently, ruminating over aspects of his faith. He now becomes preoccupied with his sense of failure, doubting that God can forgive him and is convinced that he must get every future decision right. He remembers the teachings of Jewish sages: 'Repent one day before you die'. Through prayer he repents again and again, spending hours each day in prayer and fasting, asking God for forgiveness. His fears focus on the minutiae of life. When he wakes in the morning, he is unsure what clothes to put on. He sees these decisions as being judged constantly by God, and he is afraid of getting things wrong. Things reach a stage where even deciding what to eat and what to say become caught up in a cycle of torment where David fears he will be condemned by God, and as a result he becomes increasingly paralysed.

Here, the CBT perspective can help. In CBT, the narrative is seen as the formulation. From this perspective, obsessive–compulsive disorder (OCD) is entirely understandable in terms of the beliefs and behaviours that drive it. Daniel is doubting his relationship with God and feels constantly judged. He feels responsible for failing both his wife and his faith. In his anxiety he keeps trying to do things right, avoiding situations where he might get decisions wrong, having to check and recheck doors and so on to make sure there have been no bad consequences for others. Doing this gives short-lived relief from anxiety, which, however, is highly reinforcing and further builds the cycle of checking and avoidance.

Daniel eventually sees his general practitioner (GP), who refers him to a local psychiatrist. He is prescribed sertraline, an antidepressant that also can be prescribed in OCD. The dose is kept high for several months. At the same time he is referred to a therapist for CBT. Daniel is able to make good use of the sessions he is offered. He comes to realise that checking and avoiding taught him the unhelpful 'rule' that these behaviours were a useful means of coping. He comes to realise that facing his fears for what they are, rather than responding by checking, avoiding or by asking over and over for forgiveness, is much more helpful. Gradually things settle down, and eventually Daniel recovers his faith, which once again acts as a support.

## Helen's story

Helen is in her mid-twenties and qualified at university a year ago with a degree in business studies. She is now working in a demanding job as assistant to a well-known publisher and has various fast-moving deadlines.

Helen remembers a happy childhood. However, she recalls that her mother was often under stress and used to have occasional panic attacks (she still suffers from anxiety). Her parents always expected her to do well at school, and even if she got a top mark, they never gave her much praise. She describes herself as having always been 'sensible' and a hard worker. Helen is close to both her parents, and chats to them on the telephone several times a week. She is physically well, but had asthma as a child. She has an inhaler she uses if she ever becomes wheezy.

At both school and university Helen would become stressed and unable to sleep before her exams. In spite of this, she got a good second-class degree, but thinks she has let herself down by failing to get a first. She attended the Christian Union at university, and finds her faith and her prayers an encouragement and helpful in her life. She feels that as a Christian she should be a good witness, being responsible, hardworking and reliable. She also has some good friends at church who she meets regularly, and she trusts and respects the local minister who she knows she can turn to if she needs.

Helen is dedicated to her job. She starts work early, has only a short lunch break and typically stays late to 'keep on top of things'. Her work involves liaising with printers and proofreaders who can be situated across different time zones. Emails come in at all times of day and night and instead of switching her smartphone off, she responds to them out of hours both at home and on holiday. Helen realises she has high standards – 'If a job is worth doing, it is worth doing well' is her core belief. She also believes that when pressures build up she must knuckle down and work harder to get through them. This has been reinforced by the implicit rules she has seen at home. Her parents keep their small house and garden immaculate and have always been concerned about appearances and what others think.

Helen loves her job, but no matter how hard she works, she keeps making small mistakes. When these happen she is very self-critical and talks to herself angrily saying 'you stupid idiot, you should have got that right. They'll think you're stupid'. As pressures mount, she starts to feel increasingly anxious and spends more and more time on documents and emails in an attempt to 'get things right' before sending them out. None of the errors she makes are seen as serious by her colleagues or her boss, who see her as doing an excellent job. However, Helen goes home late each evening feeling stressed out and exhausted; she finds it hard to relax, and she has now started to get irritable with her boyfriend Tom, making excuses not to meet him in the evening because she feels she should be working. She continues to pray, and finds that helpful, getting some Bible study notes on the Psalms and spending time looking at readings about God's peace, support and strength.

Helen is still just about coping when she goes down with a bad chest infection and worsening asthma, and is off work for 10 days. At home she lies in bed worrying about all the things she has not done, and as a result goes back to work at the first opportunity before she has fully recovered. When she returns, Helen sees nothing but undone work and imminent deadlines, realises she cannot cope and fears she will be sacked. The result is she reduces those activities that usually help her, such as listening to praise music, reading the Bible, praying each day and going to church most Sundays. As a result, she starts to feel even worse, seeing herself as failing as a Christian and letting God down.

Because Helen always likes to play down troubles and put on a good front, she hasn't told her parents how she feels and has been giving bland assurances that 'everything is fine'. When they have probed she has become irritable and shouted at her mother. She now feels guilty about that too, and doesn't want to call her back, which only adds to her guilt and sense of failure.

### Helping Helen make sense of her problems

Helen does not connect up what is happening to her, seeing instead a long list of different problems:

- 'I'll be sacked'
- 'I need to work harder to get through everything'
- 'I must get everything right'
- 'I can't cope'
- 'They'll think I'm stupid'
- 'I can't get all this done now I've been off sick'
- 'There is too much to do'
- 'I have to answer emails at home or I'll not keep up'
- 'Tom is complaining he never sees me'
- 'I can't sleep'
- 'I'm letting God down'
- 'I feel so tired'
- 'I'm losing weight and picking at food'
- 'I feel so stressed'
- 'I'm being snappy and irritable'
- 'I'm a failure in my job, and as a daughter and Christian.'

# SPIRITUALITY AND ANXIETY DISORDERS

**Life situation, relationships + practical problems**
- Recently off work ill
- Work mounting up. Pressures at home and work

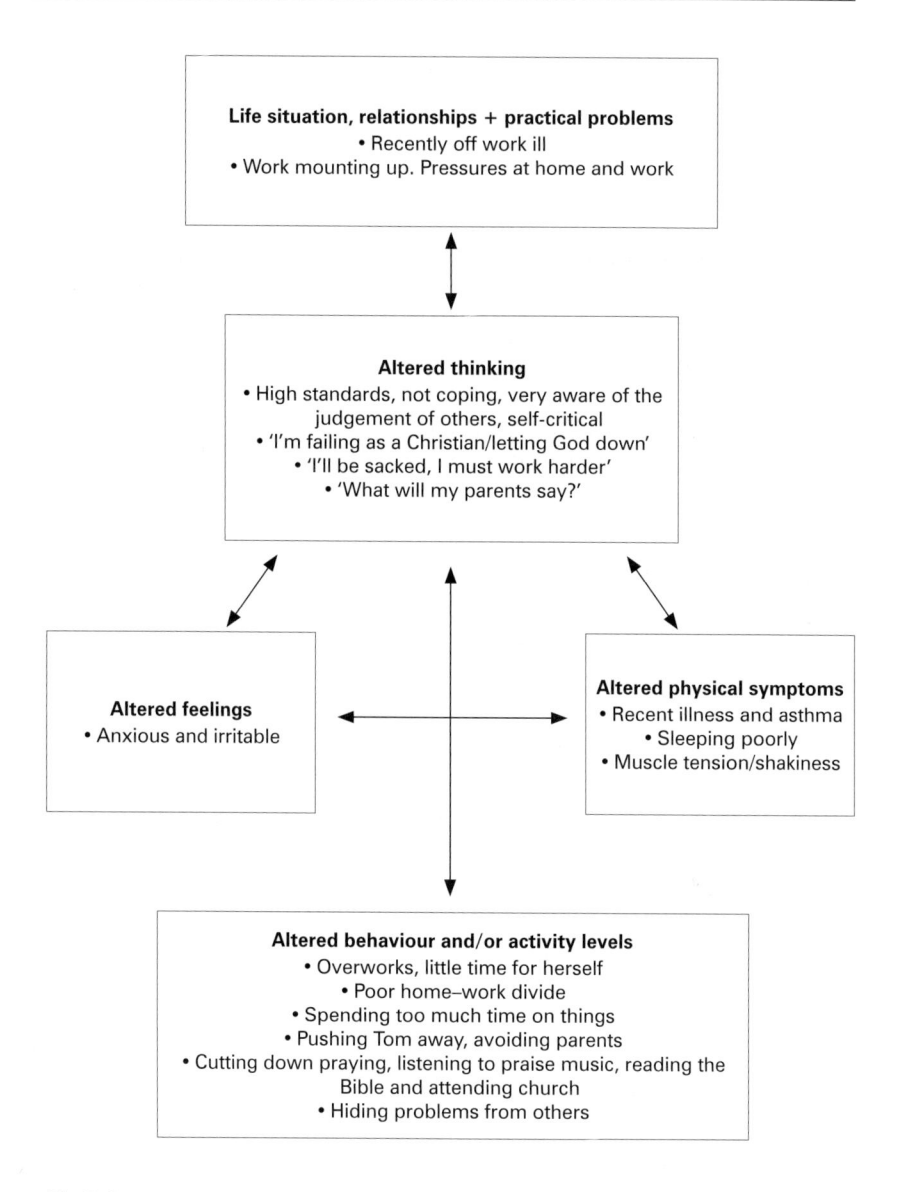

**Altered thinking**
- High standards, not coping, very aware of the judgement of others, self-critical
- 'I'm failing as a Christian/letting God down'
- 'I'll be sacked, I must work harder'
- 'What will my parents say?'

**Altered feelings**
- Anxious and irritable

**Altered physical symptoms**
- Recent illness and asthma
- Sleeping poorly
- Muscle tension/shakiness

**Altered behaviour and/or activity levels**
- Overworks, little time for herself
- Poor home–work divide
- Spending too much time on things
- Pushing Tom away, avoiding parents
- Cutting down praying, listening to praise music, reading the Bible and attending church
- Hiding problems from others

**Fig 7.2** Helen's five areas assessment.

Not surprisingly, Helen feels overwhelmed. She goes to her GP, who diagnoses generalised anxiety disorder, now coupled with exhaustion from her recent illness, and refers her for CBT.

## Helen's CBT assessment

The CBT formulation summarises the person's problems (Beck *et al*, 1979). One helpful approach to understanding the impact of anxiety is to consider the ways that it affects different areas of our life. The five areas assessment (Williams, 2013) summarises the impact of anxiety (or indeed any other problems) on five important aspects of life, and aims to be an accessible way of communicating the CBT approach (Fig. 7.2).

Each of the five areas (situation, relationship or practical problems, thinking, emotional and physical feelings, and behaviour changes) affects each other. The diagram describes a vicious circle of symptoms that only worsen how Helen feels.

There are some additional key aspects:

- What Helen thinks can affect how she feels emotionally and physically.
- What Helen thinks can affect what she does – with avoidance, or a range of responses she believes make her feel better. However, when those responses backfire, her situation is made worse.

**Table 7.1** Five areas assessment

| Area | Resources that can engender a helpful cycle |
|---|---|
| Life situation, relationships and practical problems | Helen's boyfriend is a Christian and he could help her and pray with her. The minister, friends from church and her parents are among the helpful people around. She has previously asked others to pray for her at times such as starting a new job and found that helpful. However, she realises that she has kept her problems hidden from key people (parents, Tom and friends at church, plus her boss) and needs to change this.<br>Her relationship with God is important to her and provides a sense of encouragement and hope. She could pray and ask trusted friends/minister to pray also. |
| Altered thinking | Helen's use of the Psalms and listening to praise music has previously helped her focus on things that are helpful, good and peaceful. Planning these back into her life might help her move her thoughts away from the worries onto a wider picture. |
| Altered feelings (moods or emotions) | During times of prayer, and when listening to music, Helen feels more rested and at peace. She has reduced these activities, and it may benefit her to start doing them again in a regular way. |
| Altered physical symptoms/feelings in the body | Helen remembers that in years past she attended some meditation classes in the church hall and learned a breathing technique that helped her. She could start to use that again as a regular meditation and focus to prayer. |
| Altered behaviour and/or activity levels | Helen knows that her faith is a genuine support for her. Having a pattern of daily prayer, Bible study and attending church services on a Sunday has previously helped give her life a routine that has helped. She can also choose to remind herself of God's promises for help and forgiveness. |

Although CBT aims to summarise Helen's current problems, it does not ignore the past. So the assessment also aims to make links between her current state and patterns of thinking/behaviour she has learned in the past. The approach includes beliefs and behaviour as well as relationships. In Helen's case this will importantly include her religious and spiritual values.

## How can Helen's spiritual beliefs help?

While the five areas assessment describes a downward spiral of interacting problems that are making Helen feel worse, it is also the means of identifying things that can produce a helpful cycle of recovery (Table 7.1).

The aim of CBT is to identify and build upon helpful/adaptive responses, and at the same time reduce unhelpful behaviour patterns or replace them with more helpful responses. In Helen's case, the recovery plan aims to reintroduce those important activities that she knows have helped in the past. Her CBT approach can therefore usefully incorporate faith elements that are important to her; it needs to fit with her life view – what is meaningful to her – and be consistent with her own values. These elements can be used alongside other more traditional CBT interventions focused on changing unhelpful thoughts and behaviours.

## Incorporating faith-based elements in the CBT approach

Helen's CBT therapist does not share her spiritual views, but he makes sure the work they do together can involve important aspects of Helen's own faith views. He is able to help Helen identify ways in which her anxiety has affected her faith. Helen realises she has cut down on her regular personal prayer and Bible study, and has also withdrawn from Bible study groups and attending church on Sunday. To start with, while she is still feeling stressed, she decides in the first instance to start reading the Bible every day for just 5 minutes, and to pick the encouraging Psalms in her study notes to focus on.

Over the next few weeks she starts going to church, arriving exactly on time and leaving as soon as the service ends to avoid being caught in any 'how are you' conversations. However, the service itself provides her with important support. She realises that listening to praise songs helps her relax, and she starts playing them at home and in the wind down to sleep.

After 3 weeks Helen decides to reply to a text message from her midweek group leader. She apologises for being away and says she'll aim to attend the next Wednesday. She immediately gets a text back saying she's been missed and they look forward to seeing her. On Wednesday she feels tired and decides to not go. But then she remembers from her work with the therapist on avoidance that although this might feel easiest, she will feel bad, and also others might be concerned. She stays in touch by sending a text with her apologies and says she hopes to attend the following week. She does exactly that and really enjoys the group. Others are nice towards her and supportive – providing an effective challenge to her fears that other Christians will criticise her for not being joyful and at peace all the time. In contrast, one of the leaders for whom she has great respect lets the whole group know how he had experienced stress and depression a few years back. This is a real surprise to Helen, and she is slowly able to share more about her problems and ask for prayer.

Over the next few weeks she also sees the minister and tells her how she feels. The minister says she will pray for her, and they talk about how common such issues are. The minister helps Helen realise that many of the 'Bible heroes' struggled in different ways. Some were scared, some struggled with depression or fear, others made all sorts of mistakes and yet throughout, they were loved by God. Hearing this helps Helen begin to relax. She realises she is not invincible and does not have to do everything by herself. She slowly is able to feel at peace about her situation and gradually recovers her balance at work, in her relationship and in her faith.

## Conclusions

Cognitive–behavioural therapy helps the person understand why they feel as they do, how symptoms interrelate and how they may be controlled by focusing on identifying and changing unhelpful patterns of thinking (cognitions), behaviour and relationships in ways that enable the person to make changes that help.

This chapter has focused on CBT for anxiety disorders in which spiritual/religious beliefs have played a significant part in the personal narrative. From an evidence-based perspective, it has been shown that religious/spiritual therapies can be helpful in a wide range of mental disorders (Hook *et al*, 2010), and that religiously integrated CBT has been found to be effective in depression across several faith traditions (Pearce *et al*, 2015).

Spiritual/faith aspects can readily be incorporated into CBT because they can be construed in terms of the three key elements of beliefs, behaviour and relationships, encompassing personal behaviour, and the community support from others of the same belief and God. In the narrative of Helen, she is helped to address issues that are important to her within an evidence-based framework that can incorporate spiritual values – an approach that offers hope for change in both the present and the future. The same broad approach can be used for all religious and spiritual affiliations. The key lies in identifying factors that increase helpful responses, identify and change unhelpful responses and shift extreme and unhelpful thinking to more balanced and helpful thoughts that improve how the person feels.

In summary, CBT, having demonstrated its efficacy in the treatment of secular forms of psychological distress, can also be helpfully used in the management of anxiety associated with religious and spiritual problems.

# References

Beck, A.T. (1991) Cognitive therapy as the integrative therapy. *Journal of Psychotherapy Integration*, **1**, 191–8.

Beck, A.T., Rush, J.A., Shaw, B.F., et al (1979) *Cognitive Therapy of Depression*. Guilford Press.

Fagerlin, A. (2010) Patients' knowledge about 9 common health conditions: The DECISIONS Survey. *Medical Decision Making*, **30** (suppl.): s35–52.

Hagger, M.S. & Orbell, S. (2003) A meta-analytic review of the common-sense model of illness representations. *Psychology and Health*, **18**, 141–84.

Hook, J.N., Worthington Jr, E.L., Davis, D.E., et al (2010) Empirically supported religious and spiritual therapies. *Journal of Clinical Psychology*, **66**, 46–72.

National Institute for Health and Care Excellence (2011) *Generalised Anxiety Disorder and Panic Disorder (with or without Agoraphobia) in Adults: Management in Primary, Secondary and Community Care – Quick Reference Guide*. NICE.

Pearce, M.J., Koenig, H.G., Robins, C.J., et al (2015) Religiously integrated cognitive behavioral therapy: a new method of treatment for major depression in patients with chronic medical illness'. *Psychotherapy (Chicago)*, **52**, 56–66.

Rose, D., Thornicroft, G., Pinfold, V., et al (2007) 250 labels used to stigmatise people with mental illness. *BMC Health Services Research*, **7**, 97.

Williams, C.J. (2010) *Overcoming Anxiety, Stress and Panic: A Five Areas Approach*, 2nd edn. Hodder-Arnold.

Williams, C.J. (2013) *Overcoming Depression and Low Mood*, 4th edn. Taylor & Francis/CRC Press.

Williams, C.J., Richards, P. & Whitton, I. (2002) *I'm Not Supposed to Feel Like This: A Christian Self-Help Approach to Depression and Anxiety*. Hodder & Stoughton.

CHAPTER 8

# Stories of transgression: narrative therapy with offenders

Gwen Adshead

'Nobody interrupts when the murderers talk' (Celan, 1997: p. 18).

In this chapter, I want to describe those psychological therapies that are called index offence work, that is therapeutic interventions of a psychological nature that explore the experience of causing deliberate harm to others. My experience is based on running therapy groups for men who have killed at a time when they (the perpetrators) were deemed to be mentally ill. I have also drawn on the experience of individual work with perpetrators of homicide and child abuse, especially mothers who have harmed their children.

This book has two explicit foci: the value of a narrative approach to therapeutic work and the relationship of narrative to a spiritual perspective. As previously discussed in this book, the definition of the term 'spiritual' leads to complex debates without a single 'sound-bite' answer. I, for one, am content that there is no single answer since it seems clear that the domain of 'the spiritual' encompasses a range of complex human matters that include consideration of non-material values and non-physical realities, accounts of faith and commitment, not only belief *in* but also belief *that*, as well as all the processes and practices by which we can deepen our conscious awareness of ourselves and others and come to know ourselves (Rowson, 2013). What I perceive the narrative and the spiritual to have in common is an inquiring stance that assumes that humans want to make meaning of their actions and lives, if they can; and I assume that stance is also consistent with most forms of psychotherapeutic enquiry.

I describe an approach to therapy that utilises traditional techniques (cognitive, dynamic, group) and newer metacognitive techniques such as mentalisation-based therapy (Bateman & Fonagy, 2006). In addition, our approach to index offence work draws on research into the linguistic coherence of narratives as an indicator of attachment security (Hesse, 2008). This research suggests that close attention to the language people use in therapy can reveal emotional activity and psychological processing of which the speaker may not be aware. Often the spoken word reveals the speaker's experience of agency and choice – a complex relationship between their understanding of how the choice was made and the judgement that is passed on their actions (Langer, 1991).

I will suggest that the recovery process in forensic settings involves an attempt to transform narratives of cruelty and madness into narratives of regret and hope. I say 'attempt' because there are significant obstacles to this process owing to the nature of the harm done and the stigma associated with it. I will explore some of the obstacles and the moral ambiguities associated with applying the concept of recovery to life after homicide. I hope to demonstrate parallels with traditional 'spiritual' accounts of how hearts and minds may be transformed by brokenness, suffering and despair (Rohr, 2012). Specifically, I will discuss the concept of redemption and what it might mean for people who have killed.

The patients I work with have given their permission for material from therapy to be used for teaching and research, although no historical details of any person's life are given and pseudonyms are used throughout.

## Narratives and recovery

Narrative is at the heart of the recovery and change process in mental health (Slade, 2009). Our narratives are the stories we tell of ourselves, our choices and experiences that make up our identities, as opposed to the type of information that we might use in a curriculum vitae. Over the course of a person's lifespan, narratives change and develop, being dynamic rather than fixed. Narratives are complex, layered, and integrate different perspectives of the self and social roles; they acknowledge that we may see things differently over time, and how we see ourselves may not be what others see.

The recovery movement in mental health services has emphasised the importance of narrative for a number of reasons. First, it emphasises the importance of the personal lived experience of people with mental illness or injury, as opposed to the case history record with its emphasis on diagnostic labels and the results of professional observations and investigations. Second, telling one's story has always been an important part of owning experience, as exemplified by the 12-step programme of Alcoholics Anonymous (arguably the first psychological programme to use the language of recovery). Finally, the concept of recovery implies a process of change, contrasted with fixed and categorical ways of defining people: the story of how a person lives with schizophrenia is likely to change over time, which the bald diagnosis of schizophrenia does not allow.

Narrative approaches to therapy are not new (White & Epston, 1990). Indeed, one might argue that they are ancient – that stories and myths are always about psychological change. For example, most 'quest' stories involve a transformation of the main character into a 'hero', usually after many trials and challenges (Booker, 2004). At the end of a story, most people are changed in some way: they are both literally and figuratively in a different place. In recovery narratives the story is a positive one in which a new voice is found and bad experiences are transformed into good. The following quote (from a book about alcoholism) makes the point:

> 'Narrative is not a cure, but it is a method, a path toward redemption. Redemption lies in a better understanding [...] recognising counterfeit, seeing through duplicity and resisting snares and seductions' (O'Reilly, 1997: p. 138).

And this, from a theological paper:

> 'Language can be a means of redemption, and then in some mysterious way, language is healed and healing' (Louth, 1989: p. 155).

Dan McAdams' work on narrative approaches to life change emphasises the narrative level of the personality (McAdams, 1996; McAdams & Pals, 2006). He argues that narrative reconstructions of the self are mirrors of psychological change, especially in the context of the experience of negative or traumatic events. He utilises the concept of redemption to describe the process whereby people describe surviving bad events and changing the language of a troubled or tormented self into a more hopeful, generative self: a personal identity that uses the language of hope and possibility (McAdams, 2006).

Personal narratives have been popular in non-fictional accounts of overcoming traumatic or negative events such as trauma or illness and act as a counter-perspective to professional accounts. They can be a particularly rich way to describe the process of living with mental illnesses such as depression (Styron, 1992; Solomon, 2002; Lewis, 2006) and, as McAdams suggests, 'redeem' something positive out of the negative, usually in terms of lessons learned and change of attitude to self or others.

## Narratives of offending

A particularly ancient form of story or mythic narrative is the story of the overcoming of an offending monster that threatens a community (Booker, 2004). In traditional stories, the monster is defeated or killed by the hero; the process of finding and defeating the monster is the means by which an ordinary person is transformed into a hero. In the modern world, the monster is usually a psychological monster – the monster within. One thinks here of the concept of inner demons that must be conquered before a true hero's self is discovered. Heroism is (in Walt Disney's words) a work of heart; the hero is liberated by his valiant deeds and labours that painfully bring about a positive change. Much offender rehabilitation ideology has the same vision, namely that with hard work and painful reflection a man can overcome his inner 'monster'.

Early studies of the narrative of offenders focused on their language and how they describe experience of arrest and confinement (Parker, 1969, 1990; Presser, 2004). Tony Parker was one of the first researchers to use taped and transcribed interviews that allowed the voice of a previously excluded group to be heard. Lois Presser's study of gang members in prison found that they used language that emphasised their heroic nature, and minimised their offender status. Such language is typical of neutralisation discourses (Sykes & Matza, 1957) in which what is 'neutralised' is the experience of negative feelings that might cause pain or distress in the offender such as shame, guilt, anxiety or self-reproach. Like other human beings, most offenders want to see themselves as good people who have made mistakes or been provoked into doing wrong. Psychological processes (both intrapersonal and interpersonal) that encourage the ownership of responsibility and agency for wrongdoing may be painful to experience, and generate negative affects of shame and grief that have to be endured and accommodated into an offender's sense of identity.

Professionals working with offenders in rehabilitation programmes hope that offenders who can 'own' their agency and responsibility for offending are less likely to reoffend. Although this hope intuitively accords with cultural and religious norms, there is surprisingly little research to support it. One study by Maruna (2001) does provide some empirical evidence that ownership of personal responsibility for choices made is associated with desisting from crime. Maruna examined the narratives generated by two groups of offenders, those who had desisted from crime and those who had not. The 'desisters' generated narratives of themselves that emphasised their sense of a 'previous' offending self which was not 'real'; and also used language that indicated that they experienced a sense of agency in making changes to their lives. In contrast, the 'persisters' (who continued to offend) used language that suggested that they experienced themselves in a passive way, as people to whom things just 'happened'. Maruna's work echoes research on the effectiveness of psychological therapies which found that people who had a positive experience of therapy typically described an enhanced sense of agency and effectiveness at the end of therapy (Adler et al, 2008).

## Coherence of narrative

The concept of coherence is crucial to any discussion of narrative. Narrative is essentially communicative, so it needs to engage the listener. A coherent narrative does this by being internally consistent and promoting engagement with others through the use of what the philosopher Grice (1975) calls communicative principles or conversational maxims:

1 Quality: be truthful and have evidence for what you say. Explain any apparent contradictions or reflect on them in some way with awareness.
2 Quantity: neither running on interminably nor speaking so tersely that the communicative process is lost.

3   Relevance: keeping to the subject in hand. When changing topics, licensing change with some explanation or indication of how they connect.
4   Manner: completing speech acts, use of grammar and syntax, appropriate use of imagery, metaphor and tense.

Work using Grice's conversational maxims has shown that coherent self-narratives are more common in people who have a psychologically secure sense of self (Hesse, 2008; Cassidy *et al*, 2012). Conversely, speakers who have an insecure sense of self generate narratives that are incoherent in a variety of ways. This distinction is most clearly seen in autobiographical narratives, especially narratives of early childhood attachment figures and adversity. Compared with securely attached children, insecurely attached children talk about themselves in ways that are sparse in detail and lack words for negative feelings or the personal pronoun (Cicchetti & Beeghly, 1987; Beeghly & Cicchetti, 1994).

Coherence does not mean elegant prose or flowery language: a coherent narrative is one that communicates a message with meaning in a fresh, authentic and reflective way. Here is a quote from Tim, a member of a therapy group for men who killed someone close to them:

> I feel I'm stuck in my previous age… the age I was when I did my offence… Time's passing here and there are things I'm not doing… I want to capture time with magazines and pictures to show what I was doing when I was here… What will it be like in 10 years' time? Where will we be? What will I think on my deathbed about this time?

The language communicates a lively, thoughtful voice, asking serious questions about complex human experience. The language is not complicated or extensive, but in a few well-chosen words Tim conveys his awareness of how time changes perspective, and that time is changing and moving while he is not moving in terms of his physical detention. The existential question about the end of life indicates Tim's awareness of the self-reflective process that takes place across the lifespan: that he is thinking about what he will think about himself and the meaning of his total experiences across time. He communicates a complex thought in a set of speech acts that are clear, concise and indicate a willingness to cooperate conversationally in the dialogue that is taking place in the group.

Incoherence of personal narrative is manifest in language in many different ways. Common examples include denial of distress and suffering, so that speakers idealise their past or claim to know nothing of it, or use of passive forms of verbs so that speakers are not 'actors' in their own story. Highly disorganised narratives often respond to questions with 'I can't think', as though the speaker is blanking out thought or lapsing into dissociation. Odd associations and metaphors may be present, often hinting at the experience of extremes of fear and distress.

We can compare the coherence of Tim's narrative with this excerpt from an interview with Kevin about his memories of early childhood experience.

The interviewer is asking about childhood disruptions, in this case parental divorce:

THERAPIST: Did they divorce?

PATIENT: Well I don't know if he divorced [her] or not but all I know is that he left her in a sense that he told her about his companion as he called her and to cut a long story short I blamed him for her demise because the last flicker of flame in her belly had been extinguished.

THERAPIST: What did she do when she heard?

PATIENT: Of course, yeah, after being married to [him] since childhood days, see aunts and all the rest of it, you know from back in the army days and all the rest of it, and I thought well, he's responsible for her demise, I was just grieving so much I didn't know what to do so I thought I would kill him, probably glad that he wasn't in really, he wasn't in so I got in through the back door at the side of the house and went to go and hang myself in a tree but that didn't work so I left.

Note that an incoherent narrative is not incomprehensible: it is perfectly possible to read Kevin's answers to the questions and infer what he means. However, a close look at the language of the narrative shows a variety of violations of Grice's cooperative maxims. We can notice how Kevin answers a very simple question with an elaborated answer that shifts very quickly from a factual reply to a discussion of a death, and Kevin's feelings about this. His first answer contains a beautiful but strange metaphor that does not help us understand why Kevin wants to communicate this at this point. His second answer again moves swiftly away from discussing someone's actions (which was the question) to a continuing (preoccupying?) discussion of death, his feelings about it and the remarkable linking of the experience of grief with instant thoughts of either homicide or suicide.

It is not that Kevin's narrative is 'wrong' or 'bad' but it is incoherent, because it does not complete the conversational task agreed and it leaves the listener confused about Kevin's choices, values and experience. Kevin's narratives do powerfully communicate his sense of distress, confusion and impulsive riskiness; it is perhaps of no surprise to learn that a few years after the events described above, Kevin was admitted to a secure hospital because he killed a complete stranger while in a psychotic state.

# Recovery and narrative approaches to therapy in forensic settings

Speakers who generate highly incoherent narratives of their early life are more likely to have clinical psychiatric diagnoses (Hesse, 2008) and to be actively mentally unwell. It follows therefore that recovery from periods of illness or mental disorganization is likely to be associated with increasing coherence of narrative (as suggested by Adler *et al*, 2008). At the level of linguistic detail, we might expect to hear more discussion about agency and perspective-taking (Maruna, 2001) or to find increased use of the first person pronoun (Van Staden & Fulford, 2004). Traumatic narratives are often characterised by verb tense shifts into the present tense (Pillemer *et al*, 1998), so that recovery would be associated with narrative descriptions of traumatic events that locate those events clearly in the past, without such shifts.

Here is an excerpt from a later interview with Kevin. He has been engaged in a mentalisiation-based therapy group and individual therapy for 18 months; he has also been on medication. This is his response to the same question about family disruptions in childhood:

> My grandmother died, I went to confront my grandfather with the intention of harming him, probably killing him actually at that time and it wasn't him... luckily for me and for him. I don't know what I would have done if I had got there if I had actually carried it out. Obviously I was very upset; I was really grief stricken and I tried to hang myself in the garden, I broke into the garage and got some rope and tried to hang myself... and that is what happened when someone dies, I am not talking about my index offence, I am talking about as a child.

For Kevin, this traumatic bereavement of his grandmother and his associated thoughts of suicide and homicide now seem to be firmly located in the past. He is keen to be clear with the interviewer that he wants to distinguish the death in childhood that so distressed him from the death that constitutes the index offence. He owns his violent intent then and links it to his distress that he can reflect on as being 'obvious'. There are no odd metaphors and there are clear breaks between ideas instead of run-on sentences with no gaps. Kevin reflects that he was 'lucky' not to have killed then; with the implication perhaps that he has not been so lucky since.

Die-hard materialists and cost-cutting managers with no therapeutic experience might argue that Kevin would have got better anyway with medication; and that the therapy was an expensive extra. But we (and Kevin) would argue that being able to develop a narrative like this about violence perpetration and distress is empowering for offenders. Taking responsibility for past violence and understanding the link with distress and pain enables Kevin and offenders like him to work with professionals to develop recovery strategies that may help to reduce future risk. Therapy that allows people like Kevin to develop and change personal narratives of a dreadful past is at the heart of the recovery process that applies to offenders as much as to other mental health service users (Drennan & Alred, 2013).

There are other compelling reasons why narrative therapy approaches are essential to add to the usual risk reduction programmes. First, offenders such as Kevin will be required to tell their 'story' to a variety of professionals in the rehabilitation process; and what they say about themselves and their offences will be closely scrutinized. Parole boards, multi-agency public protection panels and probation services are interested in how offenders understand their offences, the damage done and their attitudes to risk. Mentally disordered offenders in hospital are likely to stay longer if they cannot generate a story that others can understand (Dell & Robertson, 1988).

Second, many offence-related programmes in prisons and the community require individuals to describe their offence in detail in groups with other offenders who have committed the same offence. These exercises in 'telling your story' are usually time-limited, occurring once in a programme over the course of 90 min, and are usually challenged by other group members. This can be a negative experience for the person, associated with shame, stress and anxiety. Having an opportunity to develop an extended narrative in which shameful experiences are gradually explored may be experienced as less punitive, and therefore is more likely to be educational.

Third, there is evidence that committing a homicide can be a traumatic and disastrous event for the perpetrator, especially when the person killed is a family member (which is the case for the majority of victims of homicide). Rates of suicide are high for homicide perpetrators (Liettu *et al*, 2010) and the risk does not remit or reduce with time. Traumatic grief, post-traumatic stress disorder and severe depression have all been described in homicide perpetrators (Thomas *et al*, 1994; Gray *et al*, 2003; Papanastassiou *et al*, 2004), so supportive psychological therapy would seem to be indicated. Rynearson (1994) describes the use of group work for relatives of murder victims, and Hillbrand & Young (2004) pioneered the development of group therapy for parricide perpetrators. Coming to terms with the homicide perpetrator identity takes time, and can be painful and frightening; people need time for graded exposure to shame, distress and pain.

## Transformation and redemption

In forensic settings, the recovery process focuses first on helping people articulate their offender identity, and then supports a process of reflection and discussion that allows for the possibility of transformation. What is transformed is a 'cover story' (which is often mad and incoherent) into a more nuanced and thoughtful story that includes an account of agency, but also expresses regret, repentance and hope (Adshead, 2011). For example, this offender has some work to do still in respect of his offence narrative:

> I didn't kill anyone… you can dig him up and ask him if you don't believe me.

In contrast, the following excerpt suggests that Tom is actively working on his experience:

> Tom was a member of the homicide group, and was sometimes still actively psychotic in the group. On this occasion, he was audibly muttering to himself.
>
> THERAPIST *(in an enquiring tone)*: Tom, I can't hear what you are saying very well when it's a mutter.
>
> TOM *(suddenly speaking very clearly)*: I was thinking about the lady I killed and how I would like to say sorry… when I killed my mum I was mentally ill, but… there was no reason for me to kill the second lady.

This excerpt suggests that Tom had been thinking deeply about the offences he committed. Note the very interesting distinction that he makes between the two homicides and the acknowledgment that there is a difference in culpability for offences that have mental illness as their 'reason' and those that do not. Tom had not been offered individual therapy in the past because he was thought to be too psychotic to engage in such reflective work. Tom's contribution was all the more remarkable because he was one of the quieter members generally, and the therapists did not always know what he made of the experience of being in the group.

It is likely that many forensic patients will have incoherent self-narratives because of extremes of childhood adversity resulting in highly disorganised attachment systems. Kevin's first interview contained a wealth of tragic information about a very unhappy childhood in which he was regularly frightened and abandoned by parental figures. His story is similar to many offenders. It is known that histories of childhood abuse and neglect are much higher in prison and forensic populations than in the general population (Coid, 1992; Heads *et al*, 1997), and probably account for the equally high rates of insecure attachment found in these groups (see Adshead, 2003 for review). The offence narrative may be similarly disorganised and incoherent, with evidence of disturbance of language and cognitive distortions that range from the merely distorted ('The victim started it') to the frankly disordered ('I saw evil in his eyes and knew I must kill him').

Psychological therapies for offenders need explicitly to address narrative incoherence of self-narrative and offender identity as part of the recovery process. In fact, it might be said that offender patients need not so much to recover but discover a new way of being that incorporates the tragic past, yet looks to the future with realistic hope and determination (Ferrito *et al*, 2012).

## Problems with narrative approaches to therapy for offenders

I am afraid to think [of] what I have done.

Like any other treatment in medicine, psychological therapy can be associated with side-effects, including pain and short-term decline in well-being. If neutralisation discourses and incoherent narratives are a way to keep psychological pain out of consciousness, then there are bound to be anxieties about engaging in therapy that explores the past, both in relation to childhood and the offence. In our experience, this anxiety is more than the resistance of giving up a particular habit of thought, as suggested by the following quotes from the early sessions of the homicide group:

A: Therapy is like a car crash, it knocks you off course.
B: It's like asking us to take off all our clothes.
C: It's a long walk over here… like a marathon.
D: The therapists take you down roads you don't want to go.

Langer (1991) describes the intense psychological distress of Holocaust survivors who were forced to live in a universe where there was no morality and who were forced to make choices that they later deemed immoral or unacceptable. When survivors tried to speak the unspeakable or share the incomprehensible, Langer perceived fragmentation of the self, and a despair that does not fit with narrative tropes such as 'death with dignity' or 'the triumph of the human spirit'. There are moral ambiguities associated with having survived when others died or having ignored another's distress. Although Holocaust survivors and homicide perpetrators are very different in terms of innocence and guilt, nevertheless there are some similarities in the language used in oral narrative between those two groups. The perpetrators are also preoccupied with death and doubt they can be 'normal' again after having taken a life; they too wonder if they can ever be allowed to be happy in the future if their victim is not alive to do the same. Therapists likewise can be tempted to focus more on hope and strength than stay with the 'dark matter' of hopelessness and awe at the irreversibility of death.

Anxiety about homicide narratives is not confined to patients or their therapists. Other professionals involved may fear what the patients will say or what might happen when they experience psychological pain. There was considerable institutional resistance when a therapy group for men who had killed a close relative was first proposed. One psychiatrist said, 'We have not needed such a group for 150 years and we don't need one now'.

Another example of staff anxiety is revealed in an interchange between a therapist and the clinical team who were looking after a patient, Sharon, who had killed her partner in a brutal attack which took place over 3 days. Sharon started in individual therapy, but after a few weeks the therapist received a letter from the clinical team, saying: 'Please can you not talk to Sharon about her murderousness: she finds it upsetting'.

It is, of course, profoundly upsetting to talk seriously about murderousness in any context, but especially when one has taken a life. Therapists who do this work must take exquisite care with their communication skills and the words they use, and it may be that Sharon did experience her therapist 'upsetting' her. However, we might also think that something important was being turned over (literally 'upset') in Sharon's mind; perhaps the pre-offence identity and the narrative of events that had led to her admission, which (if understood) could help Sharon engage and own her identity as an offender. The process of accepting that one has done wrong is hard, and therapists do need to proceed carefully so that offenders do not impulsively turn their murderousness on themselves. Nevertheless, it is likely that the team could not bear to think about Sharon as a brutal murderer and a vulnerable woman who had suffered appalling abuse in childhood, and so wanted to close down a discussion that might make that tension explicit. Of course the tragedy is that if these therapeutic conversations do not take place in secure hospitals, it is hard to think where they could take place.

Finally, there are social anxieties about listening to offenders, and what might result if their identities as monsters are transformed into identities as protagonists in human tragedies. Knowing who and where the monsters are helps groups feel safe, and so creating monstrous identities for offenders is an important role for the media. One thinks here of a well-known UK female prisoner, convicted of killing small children, whose later (rather ordinary-looking) photographs were never used in newspapers, but only the image of her at her trial; or more recently, an article about Jon Venables (one of the two boys who killed the 2-year-old James Bulger) which was headlined with the words, 'My vile life', as if his life story and experience was fixed for all time. As one of the patients put it:

You can be an ex-bus driver, [but] you can't be an ex-murderer.

## Confession, repentance and redemption: spirituality and offenders

The themes described here are inevitably spiritual in so far as they are themes about values, choices and the morality of good and evil. Readers from a Christian cultural background will appreciate the parallels between psychological therapy in a forensic setting as described above and the traditional Christian themes of ownership of wrongdoing, confession of that wrongdoing to another, repentance and regret for past wrongs, and commitment to change one's choices. The process of change is hard and painful, but can transform that which has been lost, distorted or that which is 'bad' into something 'good'. This transformation is redemptive in that something that was lost is found again.

Martha Ferrito carried out a qualitative analysis of narratives generated by men who have attended our homicide group (Ferrito et al, 2012). She used Dan McAdams' ideas about redemption in her analysis and found that this theme recurred in many narratives. Repeatedly, men described a wish that they could do something good for others in the future – some act that would make some recompense for the damage they had done. One man in particular poignantly expressed a wish that he might make something of himself in the future, 'so that two lives will not have been lost; and [the victim] will not have died in vain'.

Repentance and atonement are key spiritual themes in many traditional religious belief systems. We are struck at how often our patients say that they wish they could say sorry to their victims or to others and how often they express the view that they will not be able to do so because it would be too much for others to hear. We are also aware of how much they wish to be forgiven, and how impossible that seems. These profoundly spiritual themes are present in the group and raised by the members; we respond but do not ask proactively about these issues, chiefly because we are cautious about stepping outside our roles as therapists into something more associated with religious roles. We see ourselves as companions for these men as they walk a Via Dolorosa – companions who might help them bear their burdens but cannot take them away completely.

## Conclusions

My experience of listening to the narratives of offenders is that there can be a process of transformation from an incoherent 'cover story' to more coherent narrative of tragedy, regret and hope. This transformation takes time and needs reflective, secure thinking spaces where people who have done terrible things can learn to trust enough to say what could not previously be safely spoken. Such therapy needs therapists who are trained and ready to listen to what the offenders have to say, in their own time and in their own way. Therapists have to be acute listeners for the small shifts in narrative emphasis, tone or metaphors that indicate shifts in perspective, coherence or agency. The work of discovering a new identity after a tragedy finds an echo in that great 14th-century work of Christian mysticism, *The Cloud of Unknowing*:

> 'not what Thou art, or hast been, sees God with his merciful eye, but what thou wouldst be' (Anonymous, 1922: p. 108).

## Acknowledgements

The work that allowed me to write this chapter would not be possible without the help and support of kind and thoughtful colleagues. I would like to acknowledge here my co-therapists: Peter Aylward, supervisor, who has written a rich and thought-provoking book about homicide (Aylward, 2012) and Dr Estelle Moore, whose pioneering vision of recovery in forensic settings (Moore & Drennan, 2013) made the group possible.

## References

Adler, L.J., Skalina, L. & McAdams, D. (2008) The narrative reconstruction of psychotherapy and psychological health. *Psychotherapy Research*, **18**, 719–34.

Adshead, G. (2003) Three degrees of security. In *A Matter of Security: Attachment Theory and Forensic Psychiatry and Psychotherapy* (eds F. Pffafflin & G. Adshead): pp. 147–66. Jessica Kingsley.

Adshead, G. (2011) The life sentence: narrative approaches to the group therapy of offenders. *Group Analysis*, **44**, 175–95.

Anonymous (1922) *A Book Of Contemplation The Which Is Called The Cloud Of Unknowing, In The Which A Soul Is Oned With God*. John M. Watkins. Available at: http://www.catholicspiritualdirection.org/cloudunknowing.pdf (accessed 27 January 2016).

Aylward, P. (2012) *Understanding Dunblane and Other Massacres: Forensic Studies of Homicide, Paedophilia and Anorexia*. Karnac.

Bateman, A. & Fonagy, P. (2006) *Mentalization-Based Treatment for Borderline Personality Disorder: A Practical Guide*. Oxford University Press.

Beeghly, M. & Cicchetti, D. (1994) Child maltreatment, attachment and the self-system: emergence of an internal state lexicon in toddlers at high social risk. *Development and Psychopathology*, **6**, 5–30.

Booker, C. (2004) *The Seven Basic Plots: Why We Tell Stories*. Continuum.

Cassidy, J., Sherman, L.J. & Jones, J.D. (2012) What's in a word? Linguistic characteristics of Adult Attachment Interviews. *Attachment & Human Development*, **14**, 11–32.

Celan, P. (1997) *Wolf's Bean* (transl. M. Hamburger). Delos Press.

Cicchetti, D. & Beeghly, M. (1987) Symbolic development in maltreated youngsters: an organisational perspective. *New Directions in Child Development*, **36**, 47–68.

Coid, J. (1992) DSM-III diagnosis in criminal psychopaths: a way forward. *Criminal Behaviour and Mental Health*, **2**, 78–94.

Dell, S. & Robertson, G. (1988) *Sentenced to Hospital: Offenders in Broadmoor*. Oxford University Press.

Drennan, G. & Alred, D. (2013) Recovery in forensic mental health settings. In *Secure Recovery: Approaches to Recovery in Forensic Mental Health Settings*. Routledge.

Ferrito, M., Vetere, A., Adshead, G., et al (2012) Life after homicide: accounts of recovery and redemption of offender patients in a high security hospital – a qualitative study. *Journal of Forensic Psychiatry & Psychology*, **23**, 327–44.

Gray, N.S., Carman, N.G., Rogers, P.E., et al (2003) Post-traumatic stress disorder caused in mentally disordered offenders by the committing of a serious violent or sexual offence. *Journal of Forensic Psychiatry and Psychology*, **14**, 27–43.

Grice, H.P. (1975) Logic and conversation. In *Syntax and Semantics* (eds P. Cole & J.P. Morgan). Vol. 3: Speech acts: pp. 41–58. Academic Press.

Heads, T., Taylor, P. & Leese, M. (1997) Childhood experiences of patients with schizophrenia and a history of violence: a special hospital sample. *Criminal Behavior and Mental Health*, **7**, 117–30.

Hesse, E. (2008) The Adult Attachment Interview. In *Handbook of Attachment*, 2nd edn (eds J. Cassidy & P. Shaver): pp. 552–98. Guilford Press.

Hillbrand, M. & Young, J.L. (2004) Group psychotherapy for parricides: the Genesis Group [article in English]. *Forensische Psychiatrie und Psychotherapie Werkstattschriften*, **11**, 89–97.

Langer, L.L. (1991) *Holocaust Testimonies: The Ruins of Memory*. Yale University Press.

Lewis, G. (2006) *Sunbathing in the Rain: A Cheerful Book about Depression*. Harper Perennial.

Liettu, A., Mikkola, L., Säävälä, H., et al (2010) Mortality rates of males who commit parricide or other violent offense against a parent. *Journal of the American Academy of Psychiatry and the Law Online*, **38**, 212–20.

Louth, A. (1989) Augustine on language. *Literature and Theology*, **3**, 151–8.

Maruna, S. (2001) *Making Good: How Ex-Convicts Reform and Rebuild Their Lives*. American Psychological Association.

McAdams, D.P. (1996) Personality, modernity and the storied self: a contemporary framework for studying persons. *Psychological Inquiry*, **7**, 295–321.

McAdams, D.P. (2006) *The Redemptive Self: Stories Americans Live By*. Oxford University Press.

McAdams, D.P. & Pals, J.L. (2006) A new big five: fundamental principles for an integrative science of personality. *American Psychologist*, **61**, 204–17.

Moore, E. & Drennan, G. (2013) Complex forensic case formulation in recovery-oriented services: some implications for routine practice. *Criminal Behaviour and Mental Health*, **23**, 230–40.

O'Reilly, E.B. (1997) Sobering Tales: Narratives of Alcoholism and Recovery. Cited in *Turns in the Road: Narrative Studies of Lives in Transition* (eds. A. Lieblich, R.E. Josselson & D. McAdams): pp. 129–49. American Psychological Association (2001).

Papanastassiou, M., Waldron, G., Boyle, J., et al (2004) PTSD in a mentally ill perpetrator of homicide. *Journal of Forensic Psychiatry & Psychology*, **15**, 66–75.

Parker, T. (1969) *The Twisting Lane: Some Sex Offenders*. Hutchinson.

Parker, T. (1990) *Life After Life: Interviews with Twelve Murderers*. Secker & Warburg.

Pillemer, D., Desrochers, M., Ebanks, C. (1998) Remembering the past in the present: verb tense shifts in autobiographical memory narratives. In *Autobiographical Memory: Theoretical and Applied Perspectives* (eds C. Thompson, D.J. Herrmann, J.D. Read, *et al*): pp. 145–62. Lawrence Erlbaum.

Presser, L. (2004) Violent offenders, moral selves: constructing identities and accounts in the research interview. *Social Problems*, **51**, 82–102.

Rohr, R. (2012) *Falling Upward: A Spirituality for the Two Halves of Life*. SPCK Publishing.

Rowson, J. (2013) *Taking Spirituality Seriously*. Social Brain.

Rynearson, T. (1994) Psychotherapy of bereavement after homicide. *The Journal of Psychotherapy Practice and Research*, **3**, 341.

Slade, M. (2009) *Personal Recovery and Mental Illness*. Cambridge University Press.

Solomon, A. (2002) *The Noonday Demon*. Vintage.

Styron, W. (1992) *Darkness Visible: A Memoir of Madness*. Vintage Books.

Sykes, G. & Matza, D. (1957) Techniques of neutralization: a theory of delinquency. *American Sociological Review*, **22**, 664–70.

Thomas, C., Adshead, G. & Mezey, G. (1994) Traumatic responses to child murder. *Journal of Forensic Psychiatry*, **5**, 168–76.

Van Staden, C.W. & Fulford, K.W. (2004) Changes in the use of the first person pronouns as possible linguistics markers of recovery. *Australian and New Zealand Journal of Psychiatry*, **38**, 226–32.

White, M. & Epston, D. (1990) *Narrative Means to Therapeutic Ends*. W.W. Norton.

CHAPTER 9

# Narratives of transformation in psychosis

Isabel Clarke with Katie Mottram, Satyin Taylor[†] and Hilary Pegg

Narrative is powerful. It creates selves. It creates cultures. It weaves the context of our lives and experiences. Where those experiences lead beyond consensual reality, as with both the psychotic and the mystical, the narrative that contextualizes them is particularly striking. Our society is inclined to pathologise this facet of human experience. Satyin and Katie, whose accounts follow, are, like me, involved in developing and running the Spiritual Crisis Network (www.spiritualcrisisnetwork.org.uk), an organization that offers a hopeful and a spiritual narrative for those going through disturbing and destabilising periods in their life. Hilary is in sympathy with the aims of the Spiritual Crisis Network and is an important contributor to a supportive Yahoo email list with the same theme. Their narratives illustrate how even the darkest of times can herald transformation. My own interest in this is as a clinical psychologist with over 20 years' practice in psychiatric rehabilitation and for the past 10 years working in acute mental health services. Honouring the narratives brought by the service users and developing a therapeutic approach that incorporates their transformative potential is central to my practice.

All three personal contributions describe major breakdowns involving the psychiatric services. For Satyin this meant a long period in hospital and for Hilary a number of hospital stays. Satyin and Katie now see their 'episodes' as behind them and are forging new lives with confidence. Hilary is still recovering from her last, most disturbing, episode and for her there is a sense that the journey is not finished. Two of the contributors were given diagnoses at different times, including schizophrenia and bipolar disorder. Katie has never received a formal diagnosis. However, the approach described in this chapter is not diagnosis specific; it has been put to the test over 10 years in the National Health Service (NHS) mental healthcare (mostly in-patient) and with the full range of presentations expected in such a service.

---

[†]Satyin was known as Jim before being ordained into the Triratna Buddhist Order.

All three contributors regard their experiences as ultimately narratives of transformation rather than narratives of illness. We are passionate about offering the perspective described here to others who are going through the same, potentially including anyone whose life crisis results in their losing touch with consensual reality, or whose vulnerability means that they exist permanently in that state, and who are customarily given a psychiatric diagnosis of psychosis. However, we do recognise that this approach is controversial, and also concede that in the case of individuals who have long adapted to psychosis it is likely that potential for transformative growth has been lost.

I will first let Katie, Satyin and Hilary speak for themselves, then draw together some of the characteristics of their narratives into a framework that helps to make the link between opening to another dimension and transformation. I conclude with significant current research pointing those of us working in mental health towards a new and more positive narrative, and how service developments can benefit from this learning.

## *Katie*

I grew up with a skewed subconscious belief that I was only worthy of living if I was of help to others because my mum had attempted suicide when I was born, and then again when I was 17. I felt somehow responsible and as soon as I was old enough, I threw myself into mainstream psychiatry to protect myself with knowledge to prevent 'madness' happening to me. The more I learned, the more confused I became, as what I was learning about didn't feel authentic with my soul. Battling to understand resulted in years of feeling inadequate, depressed, and a heavy sense that in order to fit in with a reductionist approach, I had to pretend to be someone I was not.

Holding a 'professional' diagnostic view of psychosis and having witnessed my mother being compulsorily detained and given electroconvulsive treatment (she had claimed to be possessed by a spirit, believing herself to be a 'healer') I was petrified that the same would happen to me. My mum had been diagnosed with schizoaffective disorder and was now suffering badly from the side-effects of medication.

In 2008 I could no longer maintain my façade of being 'okay' and experienced a mental breakdown. Various traumatic life events took their toll on my already fragile sense of self and I made a serious attempt on my own life. Nothing made sense and living seemed futile. Petrified, knowing I was following in my mother's footsteps, I avoided seeking help, knowing where that would lead. I worked in mental healthcare, yet I could not trust the system to provide the support I so desperately needed; it made me feel like a hypocrite.

Then, in March 2012 my belief system about mental illness, the world and my place in it changed literally overnight. During a meditation I experienced a profound breakthrough; the awareness being a soul, I awoke from a state of merely existing as someone who had a mountain of self-doubt to a sense of knowing that I could be anyone I wanted to be. I could reclaim the control of my life I had been longing for but which before that moment I never believed I could have. An absolute sense of pure peace washed over me and I felt that I was totally connected to everything and everyone in the world. I had no sense of anger or fear; everything was taken over by clarity of perspective, acceptance and understanding. At that moment every piece of the jigsaw of my life made complete sense and I had not one regret, I just knew that every crisis had happened to bring me to this moment of strength. My mind had been blessed with a glimpse of another level of consciousness and it would never be the same again. My soul knew that I'd had access to the Universal consciousness, and at this time could freely communicate with spirit. It was an ineffable, amazing experience.

The irony was that having worked within the mental health system for over 12 years, my educated 'logical' brain told me I was psychotic and having delusions of grandiosity. My energy levels at the time were unbounded, and I also feared that I was manic. This chasm of comprehension between my soul and my mind threw me into panic and confusion. Continuing my 'normal' daily life without speaking about what I was experiencing at a deeper level was a real challenge, but I feared that if I told anyone who I worked with about my experience, I might end up being hospitalised.

At the same time I suddenly realised that my mum too had been experiencing a spiritual awakening, but not understanding it. I aided the resulting cycle of crisis through my part in getting her detained, unable to understand her behaviour at the time. She had spoken about getting 'messages' from spirit and being able to predict the future, and I had brushed this off as mad ramblings. Now I recognized our experiences as similar.

Over the past 2 years I have spoken openly to mum about spirituality and acknowledged her own interpretation of her experiences. After nearly 40 years of living in an emotionally frozen state, this different narrative has been the only thing that had started to bring her out of her negative belief pattern that she is crazy and worthless. Unfortunately mum's inability to process the emotional side of her trauma, her consequent lack of self-confidence following years of receiving such negative prognoses, and the absence of any appropriate support for her within mainstream services owing to a lack of understanding about this phenomena, sees her continue to be trapped in a cycle of fear and silence.

Now I very much see facing the pain as an intrinsic part of our evolutionary process. I consider myself to be hugely lucky. Despite my doubting logical brain, I had the strength of character to listen to my soul, which led me to find a group of people in the UK Spiritual Crisis Network who understood the phenomena of spiritual emergence.[1] With the stability of this conceptual framework, to make sense of my experiences and allow natural evolution and integration was like coming home – the opposite of seeing psychosis as a destructive illness. I am now more able to be a 'silent witness' to my emotions, rather than letting them control me, and I have a much more positive belief system. I know that I am on a life-long journey of learning, one I enjoy and appreciate.

This positive frame of reference in which to make sense of my experience has both helped me and given me the belief that I can make a positive difference to others. I am now working in collaboration with the peer-supported Open Dialogue pilot project, and as one of three inaugural directors for the International Spiritual Emergence Network am able to provide valuable insight into this different perspective thanks to my personal experience. I have also published a memoir to inspire hope in others who may be suffering. My ultimate mission is to help transform the mental health system into one that is more positive, progressive and open-minded.

---

1. For a discussion of the phenomenon of spiritual emergence, see Crowley (2006).

## Satyin

Growing up nominally Christian and an apparently natural pacifist, after introverted teenage years I blossomed socially at university. I also started to smoke cannabis, enjoying my own company without a sense of missing out and steeping myself more and more deeply in the music I loved. It also seemed to open me up in an unexpected way.

During the second year of my psychology degree in 1994, aged 20, I had a 'prodromal' couple of weeks of seemingly increased functioning when things apparently 'made sense'. This culminated one evening when I found myself writing a 'stream of consciousness', for exactly 4 hours. Memorably, the word 'nirvana' appeared unbidden very strongly in my mind. I was clear something different or odd was going on, so I turned to the question of the existence of God, saying to myself 'God, if you exist give me a sign'. News of the suicide of Kurt Cobain of the band Nirvana, unusual confidence in acquiring cannabis and further coincidences led to my declaring to the household: 'I think I'm Jesus'. I remember trying to convince them that something significant was happening spiritually in the universe, pointing to a TV soap opera on in the background as evidence of this.

The following days brought a series of many fascinating experiences and 'coincidences'. Increasingly my mind was racing; I was seeing things differently and recognized the possibility of 'illness' from my abnormal psychology studies. I certainly did require support, and with encouragement I went to my university general practitioner and was repeatedly assessed until I found myself tucked up in bed, informally admitted to an adult acute [psychiatric] ward.

While my unusual ideas were cause for concern, my family found it tremendously distressing to see me so sensitive to the antipsychotic medications being tried out on me. Side-effects meant one day my dad having to help me to walk; I was experiencing lockjaw, slurred speech and major stiffness – basically a dribbling wreck. At one time, my father cried, wondering if he would ever get his son back to normal. Yet I've never felt anger towards the system, I knew it was doing what it thought best.

None of the antipsychotics took away the unusual experiences, the coincidences or targeted the 'grandiose' way I had made sense of my experience. Whether things shifted naturally or because of the lithium that was eventually prescribed is unclear.

During my lengthy hospitalization I had been aware of positives: a new openness to Nature, unaccustomed skill at golf putting and spontaneous compassion. Alas, all dropped away as I got 'well'. Spiritual grandiosity was replaced by cringing embarrassment after discharge. I came down with a bump during a depressed summer, followed by successful autumn re-entry into academic life with completion of my degree and avoidance of cannabis. I did not conceal my story – a helpful lack of repression – but I felt that what had been a tremendously significant time for me was now written off as simply an illness. I moved from volunteering on the ward where I had been a patient to an occupational therapy assistant post in 1997.

In 2000 I was lucky enough to find out about and get support to attend the first of two conferences on psychosis and spirituality (Clarke, 2010a), affording me an opportunity to meet others who had had similar experiences as well as open-minded professionals who were interested in meaningful ways of understanding unusual experience. This initiated a period of revaluation of my formative meaningful experiences rather than cutting them off as illness, as usually happens.

I successively got into yoga, meditation and Buddhism. In 2004 on a Buddhist retreat, confident I would not be troubled by such strong experiences again, I saw a woman with whom I felt a most unusual tangible energy connection across the shrine room. When we spoke there seemed an instant strong connection, and we acknowledged this. I went to bed thinking 'I've met my partner, what was all the fuss about, that was straightforward'. However, this very significant relationship brought with it experiences like those of 10 years before: sleeplessness, strong energy rising and needing to write. I snapped out of the speeding mind into a sense of expansive peace and began trying to make sense of it. Having been going to Buddhist classes and retreats for 9 years I jumped to a conclusion; given the difference in consciousness I was experiencing, I announced to my partner to be that I must be 'enlightened'!

I was lucky enough to get support from people who recognized the concept of spiritual emergency,[2] who gave me pertinent advice and validation. It was important that I could find a way to make sense of, and integrate, the experience. I knew that this was a deeply meaningful experience for my personal growth. My knowledge of Buddhism and 'the hero's journey'[3] also gave me support and a positive conceptualisation of what I was going through.

As I write this narrative of my transformation, I am travelling across Europe on sabbatical from my NHS role working with psychosis, to begin a 4-month intensive ordination retreat. It is my chosen way to build the optimal conditions for gaining insight into the true nature of 'reality'. As a result of my experiences, the challenge of transcending the 'conditioned mind' is no longer an abstract concept. I know other modes of operating are possible.

## Hilary

I have had three psychoses or episodes of connecting beyond myself. The first occurred soon after my mother died and at a time when my sister was pronounced to have terminal cancer. One day in the garden a voice spoke through me saying 'my name is Al Alal, I am from the Institute of Joseph of Arimathea and I have come to help you heal your sister'. In the end Al Alal told me he was in error and that he was being taken to another part of the spirit world. From that point, things started getting bizarre. I was informed that I was attached to an aeroplane flying overhead by a chord. My husband called the doctor and a voice speaking through me said 'I am a charismatic pilot, will you please send this woman to hospital'. From the doctor's perspective, it was me who was talking but as far as I was concerned it was not my voice. I spent about a month in the hospital being visited by a variety of spirits. A spirit named Pelegeia did automatic writing with me. The episode resolved when some 'spirit doctors' arrived and told me to release the spirits attached to me by letting them jump off my tongue into a glass of water.

Before I had this experience, which was the most extraordinary thing that had ever happened in my life, I was what I would term a middle-of-the-road Christian. Now I feel open to a whole lot of beliefs, channelling, near-death

---

2. Spiritual emergency and spiritual emergence are distints phases in the process outlined by Grof & Grof (1991).
3. The concept of hero's journey is discussed in Campbell (2008).

experiences, spirit attachment and reincarnation. Rather than seeing it as an illness, I experienced this time as an awakening to new possibilities.

Two years later I had another episode in which I was told by voices (not my own) that I was to press the button that would set off all the nuclear arsenals in the world. I heard other voices doubting that I could do such a thing, but they were informed 'I had been trained'. I felt my body being moved. I was told I was the second coming of Jesus. I met God and played word games with him. I was told that I had been made into a perfect human being, though life would knock the corners off, and that a tape was being made of my life. I was told that everything in life had been perfectly planned and that everyone would be rewarded or punished according to their deserts. When I later read about karma I was amazed at the similarity. I was also asked what I wanted to do with my life and I said I wanted to stay exactly where I was, among people with mental health problems. I even remember ordaining myself.

These experiences, dismissed as meaningless by the hospital staff, inspired me to communicate my new perspective and heralded a period when I became very active. I flew up to Dundee to a conference on spirituality in mental health and following this attended two 'revisioning mental health' conferences in Stroud that marked the beginning of the Spiritual Crisis Network. I had come across the Royal College of Psychiatrists' Spirituality and Psychiatry Special Interest Group and corresponded with Dr Alan Sanderson about the nature of spirit release. I was so intrigued by this I trained in hypnotherapy and went to two conferences in London and an introductory workshop on releasing spirits. I even got my local council to part-fund my trip.

I undertook research into the work of chaplains in mental health services, gaining an MSc. A group of us put on a conference at our local trust on spirituality and mental health. I found a psychiatrist who would help me wean myself off psychiatric medication. I was becoming an evangelist for spirituality and psychosis. It was only then that I discovered the darker side, and the potential dangers of being open to this other way of experiencing.

In a third episode, I was told that I had discovered the truth about the universe and would be taken to a higher plane. Then I found myself on the floor being told to come back down to Earth and take human form quickly as I had nearly 'blown my cover'. I assumed I was an alien of some sort. I believed that my husband had married me in order to protect the public from discovering my identity. This was a frightening psychosis in which I was convinced that a terrorist group had penetrated my brain and were about to kill me. I believed the bungalow I was living in had been burned to the ground and the room I was in had been transported to another part of the universe. I had come off my medication at this time and I decided to go back on it to prevent further events happening.

For me, these episodes have been, in part, a transformative experience. While they have widened my belief system and opened me to new vistas, having a bad 'trip' was plain frightening. However, I do not regret them. After two deaths in close proximity, leaving me without a family, something needed to 'give'.

I am still working with my local mental health trust, highlighting the link between spirituality and psychosis, but I have lost the confidence to travel and never did take up spirit release therapy. This loss of confidence may be temporary, who knows, for I am on a journey. In my own mind, my faith in something bigger than myself has been enhanced and I am quite ready to believe that I had both a psychosis and a spirit attachment.

## Wider perspectives

These three accounts have elements in common that point to a way of making sense of a breakdown; of departure from shared reality and problems with functioning, which honours its transformative potential. All three can be recognized as belonging to a group of people that may be referred to as 'high schizotypes'. This is an important concept when seeking to normalize anomalous experiencing. Schizotypy is understood here as a dimension of normality and is to be distinguished from schizotypal personality disorder, a diagnosis that has little bearing on this concept. As used here, schizotypy signifies ease of access to 'non-ordinary experiencing', and aims to bring such experiences (which may attract the label of psychosis) within the compass of normality.

The body of schizotypy research conducted over decades by Claridge and his collaborators (Claridge, 1997, 2010) explores the dimension of human experience represented by openness to the unusual and the anomalous that lie beyond consensual reality. Though the predominant association for this vulnerability is psychotic breakdown, schizophrenia and so on, the body of research makes a clear association with the valued attributes of creativity and spirituality as well. The fact that Katie's mother was diagnosed with psychosis underlines that this trait does have a physical, heritable substrate, which nevertheless does not need to be understood in a reductionist way. Katie was able to extend her re-evaluation of the experience to her mother. These experiences opened horizons to take in previously excluded spiritual perspectives, involving stepping out of a normal, restricted sense of self into a place where the self was less defined, and sometimes felt to be supremely important. Hilary thought she was an alien on a mission and Satyin thought he was Jesus or had become enlightened. The lack of a safe boundary can bring fear, destabilisation and danger as Hilary experienced most strongly in her third episode, but equally it can open the way to heightened perception and attunement to synchronicities.

A sense of constriction or incompleteness prior to this opening is a common theme. Satyin had been unconfident, Katie had felt responsible for her mother's woes and Hilary had experienced multiple losses. The role that psychotic breakdown played in resolving their various difficulties can be seen in terms of Mike Jackson's 'problem-solving' model of psychosis (Jackson, 1997; Jackson, 2010). Jackson argues that this other dimension of experience opens up when normal life has reached an impasse and becomes a way forward, particularly for high schizotypes. This can enable the individual to draw on resources that were previously beyond their reach, hence the transformative potential. However, the need to protect against the vulnerability this engenders can lead to a vicious circle of getting lost in a psychotic world and becoming trapped in pathology, leading to isolation.

I have written elsewhere on how these phenomena can be understood in terms of neural processing (Clarke, 2008a, 2010b, 2013). In summary, the more recent evolutionary verbal faculty serves to filter our perceptions; by default, the rest of the brain organizes relationship, emotion and experience. Together they share control, with a capacity to desynchronize in certain circumstances, but neither is 'the boss' (Teasdale & Barnard, 1993; Barnard 2003). According to Teasdale & Barnard's interacting cognitive subsystems model of cognitive architecture, the verbal, propositional subsystem gives us our separateness and grasp of detail; the default, implicational subsystem manages relationship and emotion. When the implicational dominates, we lose the certainty of individual selfhood, leading to confusion about the boundaries of the self. With no means of monitoring between the genuine and illusory, this state can lead to persecutory synchronicities and false certainties. However, it can also open a person to genuine connection with God and the universe so characteristic of mystical experience. In contrast to everyday living, which is ruled by the logic of either/or, this state is governed by the paradoxical logic of both/and, as religious writings the world over have reflected.

While what has been said above could be regarded as speculative, recent lines of research suggest a line of continuity between psychosis and psychosis-like experiences that never progress to diagnosable illness (van Os *et al*, 2009; Linscott & van Os, 2013). Linscott & van Os conclude:

> 'Emphasis on symptomatology (actual experience as opposed to disorder class) would reduce the risk of stigmatization and facilitate the identification of proximal antecedents of distress, thereby providing a more salient, amenable target for monitoring and intervention' (p. 1145).

Research into symptoms experienced positively (Sanjuan *et al*, 2004; Jenner *et al*, 2008; Jackson *et al*, 2010) sheds further light. Jackson and colleagues conclude that 'Promoting a positive self-concept and connecting with communities who value and accept voice-hearing experiences may be particularly important' (Jackson *et al*, 2010: p. 487). The most significant body of research is the 'need for care' strand in which Emmanuelle Peters (King's College London) is prominent. Looking at groups of people with exactly comparable 'symptoms', it has been shown that the outcome is better where people have found a non-medical and essentially benign way of making sense of their anomalous experiences (Brett *et al*, 2007, 2009, 2014; Heriot-Maitland *et al*, 2012; Marks *et al*, 2012). The overall conclusion of these studies reinforces the importance of a social and cognitive context that provides hopeful and non-stigmatizing meaning for such experiences, even where they are very distressing and severely affect functioning. Spiritual conceptualisations come out particularly well. Taken together with epidemiological evidence showing that traditional societies with a less rigidly medical approach to schizophrenia show better outcome (Warner 2004, 2007), this evidence should occasion reflection for those of us who work in mental healthcare.

The concern of this chapter has been with a way of experiencing open to all human beings but more often accessed by high schizotypes. This has been the territory of saints and mystics; they too encountered terror as well as ecstasy, their experiences were frequently preceded by illness or transition, and their day-to-day functioning was often supported by a community when compromised. Many of these individuals were looked up to for the wisdom they derived from their journey (Clarke, 2008a). This way of experiencing can also arise in more profoundly disabling forms of major mental illness not identified in the examples given here. In such cases medicalization, or the stigma that may attach, cannot always be avoided but it is still possible to find ways of promoting a positive concept of self amidst the experience and to offer hope and meaning.

Those who enter this other way of experiencing can easily lose their 'selves'. In this magical and dangerous liminal state, anything is possible and it can go either way. The research quoted so far, and the experiences of Katie, Satyin and Hilary illustrate that the course of the 'illness' is powerfully influenced by how people make sense of such experiences, in turn shaped by those around them.

As the psychologist in an acute service (hospital and crisis resolution and home treatment teams), I have been concerned to make use of this potential for growth and healing. Cognitive–behavioural therapy (CBT) for psychosis can embrace mindfulness as a way of enabling the individual to gain distance between themselves and their disturbing experiences. A key factor promoting a benign outcome is the ease with which the individual can move backwards and forwards at will between 'unshared' (psychotic) and 'shared' reality. The skill of mindfulness can facilitate this movement because it can create distance between the experience and the experiencer. The growing evidence for the efficacy of CBT for psychosis by incorporating mindfulness demonstrates this (Chadwick *et al*, 2009; Dannahy *et al*, 2011).

I therefore developed a programme for delivery within the acute service called 'The What is Real and What is Not' group (Clarke, 2010c, 2013), which takes as its norm the human facility to access apparent 'other realities'. We started by looking at the spectrum of openness to unusual experiencing (schizotypy) in its positive and negative aspects. By exploring recognition of 'unshared' as opposed to 'shared' reality, it was possible to honour the positive aspects of vulnerability to this state, at the same time facing up to its problems and dangers. Spiritual aspects could be validated while also sounding a note of caution. Pointing out that 'unshared reality' is governed by a logic of 'both/and' proved useful in dealing with convictions of specialness. Indeed, this concept was usually understood quite easily by the group.

Brainstorming with the participants on the characteristics of shared and unshared reality usually produced 'frightening and lonely' but 'buzzy' for the unshared state, whereas shared reality was identified as safer, more controllable but 'boring'. This perspective provided the foundation for encouraging participants to face up to unshared reality and to learn skills such as mindfulness to manage it.

Once the group were prepared to look more dispassionately at their experiences, and let go both of the desire to 'seal over' and dismiss them or to accord them too great importance, they were in a better place to learn the skills to manage them. The role of mindfulness in enabling someone to gain distance and manage the necessary transition from 'unshared' to 'shared' reality has already been mentioned. Arousal management is another key skill. Symptomatic experiences are more accessible at times of high stress and arousal, when simple techniques such as relaxation breathing can be of benefit. Less recognised is the role of low arousal in increasing vulnerability to symptomatic experiences; hypnogogic states and the popular pastime in hospitals of looking at the TV without really watching it, need to be addressed by simple, behavioural correctives.

Once participants start to feel more on top of the situation, the idea that their psychosis might have some learning for them, the possibility of resolution of past trauma and conflict and looking out for new growth can be discussed. The manual for this group work is available online (Clarke & Pragnell, 2008).

Between 2012 and 2014 my role in an NHS trust was to reorder acute services on a holistic and therapeutic basis, along with evaluation (Durrant et al, 2007; Clarke & Wilson 2008; Araci & Clarke, 2016). This programme involves developing a narrative of ways of coping (Clarke, 2009). As well as introducing a simple psychological formulation based on 'felt sense' (Clarke, 2008*b*) and delivered under supervision, the programme is designed to involve all members of the multidisciplinary team, with training offered to all, including senior staff. The intended vision is for service users to be given a consistent message and supported through the challenge of managing overwhelming experiences; as yet it is only partially realized. The current evaluation, combining quantitative and qualitative elements, will demonstrate how far it has been achieved.

As Chair of the Psychosis and Complex Mental Health Faculty of the British Psychological Society's Division of Clinical Psychology, I am working to build alliances towards a more holistic vision of mental health problems. We are making common cause with a variety of stakeholders: service users, carers, psychiatrists (Russell Razzaque, whose new book (Razzaque, 2014) is along similar lines) and other health professionals. Our vision is to find a way of conveying a more hopeful message about mental health difficulties, in which the potential for a transformative journey can be embraced and supported. To this end, we are soon to launch an initiative called The Alliance for Re-visioning Mental Health, led by Catherine G. Lucas. Here are some suggestions for how a transformative journey for the individual may be assisted in routine mental health practice.

- Respect for experience. The experience of the mystic is respected in all cultures with the exception of reductionist scientism. Both the person with psychosis and the mystic are stepping 'beyond the self' and both deserve to be treated with respect. The propositional way of knowing is needed to engage with the everyday world of consensual reality but the implicational is equally a valid way of knowing. Without it we would be unable to navigate our relationships or to appreciate the arts.
- We must retain an open mind about the possibility of connection and influence beyond the self for those in a state of openness – whether it be a state of possession or divine influence – while keeping in mind the tricksterish, 'both/and' logic that governs this area.
- 'The feeling is real even when the story is highly suspect'. This and the concepts of shared and unshared reality are ways of talking with, and relating to, people in a psychotic state that holds the balance between the twin dangers of collusion and invalidation and that facilitates a therapeutic alliance.
- Attend to the motivational dimension. What will best persuade this individual to join the rest of us in the shared world? Motivational interviewing (Miller & Rollnick, 1991) stresses the importance of maintaining and enhancing self-esteem and self-efficacy as an essential precursor to enhancing motivation. It means taking into account the effect of a diagnosis of psychosis and all its implications for a person's self-image. Mitigating this impact enhances the likelihood of engagement and treatment adherence.
- Finally, see this person as undertaking a (probably involuntary) journey into places that most of us will not encounter and from which, following the pattern of the hero's journey into the underworld (Hartley, 2010), they have the potential to emerge stronger, and bearing gifts for the rest of us.

## Conclusions

This chapter is a challenge to those of us embedded in the prevailing system of mental healthcare. Katie, Satyin and Hilary all found that recognizing their psychosis as an actual or potential narrative of transformation enabled them to see themselves as pursuing an arduous but ultimately worthwhile path of growth. Katie, having engaged with the local NHS trust to incorporate an understanding of spiritual crisis into their spirituality policies and medical education, is now embarking on a new role as Inaugural Director for International Spiritual Emergence Network. Following Buddhist ordination Satyin has moved on from his role in psychological therapy for people with psychosis. He is now employed as a chaplain in NHS mental health services and training in the peer-supported Open Dialogue approach. Hilary sees herself as in the middle of her journey, coping with the setback to her confidence during her recent severe episode but still hopeful and working to change the paradigm through introducing the topic of spiritual narratives at the trust's regular inductions. These accounts are backed up by summary of recent research supporting the value of transformative narratives.

# References

Araci, D. & Clarke, I. (2016) Investigating the efficacy of a whole team, psychologically informed, acute mental health service approach. *Journal of Mental Health*, 8 February, doi: 10.3109/09638237.2016.1139065 [Epub].

Barnard, P. (2003) Asynchrony, implicational meaning and the experience of self in schizophrenia. In *The Self in Neuroscience and Psychiatry* (eds T. Kircher & A. David): pp. 121–46. Cambridge University Press.

Brett, C.M.C., Peters, E.P., Johns, L.C., *et al* (2007) Appraisals of Anomalous Experiences Interview (AANEX): a multidimensional measure of psychological responses to anomalies associated with psychosis. *British Journal of Psychiatry*, **191**, 23–30.

Brett, C.M.C., Johns, L., Peters, E., *et al* (2009) The role of metacognitive beliefs in determining the impact of anomalous experiences: a comparison of help-seeking and non-help-seeking groups of people experiencing psychotic-like anomalies. *Psychological Medicine*, **39**, 939–50.

Brett, C., Heriot-Maitland, C., McGuire, P., *et al* (2014) Predictors of distress associated with psychotic-like anomalous experiences in clinical and non-clinical populations. *British Journal of Clinical Psychology*, **53**, 213–27.

Chadwick, P., Hughes, S., Russell, D., *et al* (2009) Mindfulness groups for distressing voices and paranoia: a replication and feasibility trial. *Behavioural and Cognitive Psychotherapy*, **37**, 403–12.

Campbell, J. (2008) *The Hero with a Thousand Faces*, 3rd edn. New World Library.

Claridge, G.A. (1997) *Schizotypy: Implications for Illness and Health*. Oxford University Press.

Claridge, G.A. (2010) Spiritual experience: healthy psychoticism? In *Psychosis and Spirituality: Consolidating the New Paradigm*, 2nd edn (ed. I. Clarke): pp. 75–89. Wiley.

Clarke, I. (2008*a*) *Madness, Mystery and the Survival of God*. O'Books.

Clarke I. (2008*b*) Pioneering a cross-diagnostic approach founded in cognitive science. In *Cognitive Behavior Therapy for Acute Inpatient Mental Health Units; Working with Clients, Staff and the Milieu* (eds I. Clarke & H. Wilson): pp. 65–77. Routledge.

Clarke, I. (2009) Coping with crisis and overwhelming affect: employing coping mechanisms in the acute inpatient context. In *Coping Mechanisms: Strategies and Outcomes. Advances in Psychology Research* (ed. A.M. Columbus), vol. 63. Nova Science Publishers.

Clarke, I. (2010*a*) Psychosis and spirituality: the discontinuity model. In *Psychosis and Spirituality: Consolidating the New Paradigm*, 2nd edn: p. 3. Wiley.

Clarke, I. (2010*b*) Psychosis and spirituality: the discontinuity model. In *Psychosis and Spirituality: Consolidating the New Paradigm*, 2nd edn: pp. 101–15. Wiley.

Clarke, I. (2010*c*) 'What is real and what is not': towards a positive reconceptualisation of vulnerability to unusual experiences. In *Psychosis and Spirituality: Consolidating the New Paradigm*, 2nd edn: pp. 195–205. Wiley.

Clarke, I. (2013) Spirituality: a new way into understanding psychosis. In *Acceptance and Commitment Therapy and Mindfulness for Psychosis* (eds E.M.J. Morris, L.C. Johns & J.E. Oliver): pp. 160–168. Wiley-Blackwell.

Clarke, I. & Pragnell, K. (2008) *The Woodhaven 'What is real & what is not?' Group Programme'*. Woodhaven Psychological Therapies Service. Available at http://www.isabelclarke.org/docs/What_is_real_programme.pdf (accessed 6 November 2015).

Clarke, I. & Wilson, H. (eds) (2008) *Cognitive Behaviour Therapy for Acute Inpatient Mental Health Units; Working with Clients, Staff and the Milieu*. Routledge.

Crowley N. (2006) *Psychosis or Spiritual Emergence? Consideration of the Transpersonal Perspective within Psychiatry*. Royal College of Psychiatrists.

Dannahy, L., Hayward, M., Strauss, C., *et al* (2011) Group person-based cognitive therapy for distressing voices: pilot data from nine groups. *Journal of Behavior Therapy and Experimental Psychiatry*, **42**, 111–16.

Durrant, C., Clarke, I., Tolland, A., *et al* (2007) Designing a CBT service for an acute inpatient setting: a pilot evaluation study. *Clinical Psychology and Psychotherapy*, **14**, 117–25.

Grof, C. & Grof, S. (1991) *The Stormy Search for the Self*: pp. 31–33. Mandala.

Hartley, J. (2010) Mapping our madness: the hero's journey as a therapeutic approach. In *Psychosis and Spirituality: Consolidating the New Paradigm*, 2nd edn (ed. I. Clarke): pp. 227–39. Wiley.

Heriot-Maitland, C., Knight, M. & Peters, E. (2012) A qualitative comparison of psychotic-like phenomena in clinical and non-clinical populations. *British Journal of Clinical Psychology*, **51**, 37–53.

Jackson, L.J., Hayward, M. & Cooke, A. (2010) Developing positive relationships with voices: a preliminary Grounded Theory International. *Journal of Social Psychiatry*, **57**, 487–95.

Jackson, M.C. (1997) Benign schizotypy? The case of spiritual experience. In *Schizotypy. Relations to Illness and Health* (ed. G.S. Claridge). Oxford University Press.

Jackson, M.C. (2010) The paradigm-shifting hypothesis: a common process in benign psychosis and psychotic disorder. In *Psychosis and Spirituality: Consolidating the New Paradigm*, 2nd edn (ed. I. Clarke): pp. 139–55. Wiley.

Jenner, J.A., Rutten, S., Beuckens, J., *et al* (2008) Positive and useful auditory vocal hallucinations: prevalence, characteristics, attributions, and implications for treatment. *Acta Psychiatrica Scandinavica*, **118**, 238–245.

Linscott, R.J. & van Os, J. (2013) An updated and conservative systematic review and meta-analysis of epidemiological evidence on psychotic experiences in children and adults: on the pathway from proneness to persistence to dimensional expression across mental disorders. *Psychological Medicine*, **43**, 1133–49.

Marks, E.M., Steel, C. & Peters, E. (2012) Intrusions in trauma and psychosis: information processing and phenomenology. *Psychological Medicine*, **42**, 2313–23.

Miller, W.R. & Rollnick, S. (1991) *Motivational Interviewing: Preparing People to Change*. Guilford Press.

Razzaque, R. (2014) *Breaking Down is Waking Up*. Watkins Publishing.

Sanjuan, J., Gonzalez, J.C., Aguilar E.J., *et al* (2004) Pleasurable auditory hallucinations. *Acta Psychiatrica Scandinavica*, **110**, 273–8.

Teasdale, J.D. & Barnard, P.J. (1993) *Affect, Cognition and Change: Remodelling Depressive Thought*. Lawrence Erlbaum Associates.

van Os, J., Linscott, R.J., Myen-Germeys, I., *et al* (2009) A systematic review and meta-analysis of the psychosis continuum: evidence for a psychosis proneness–persistence–impairment model of psychotic disorder. *Psychological Medicine*, **39**, 179–95.

Warner, R. (2004) *Recovery from Schizophrenia: Psychiatry and Political Economy*, 3rd edn. Brunner-Routledge.

Warner, R. (2007) Review of Recovery from Schizophrenia: an International Perspective. A Report from the WHO Collaborative Project, the International Study of Schizophrenia. *American Journal of Psychiatry*, **164**, 1444–5.

CHAPTER 10

# My story: a spiritual narrative

Jo Barber

Think of a shy, obsessively studying teenager terrified of failure. Think of a solitary schoolgirl, practising the violin devotedly every break time. Think of a confused, guilt-ridden, lonely and struggling student. Think of a mute, motionless patient on a psychiatric ward, in despair. Think of a person coping independently, doing voluntary work. Think of someone feeling fulfilled and happy for the first time in life.

All these things describe my life at different stages.

I have been a mental health service user for 30 years with many ups and downs. Here I write my journey, through illness to comparative wellness, as a 'spiritual' narrative.

In common with most people (Rogers *et al*, 2002), my spiritual experiences have always been in a state of flux. Sometimes my faith has seemed more important and sometimes the music, sometimes both at once. Sometimes one or other or both have been positively unhelpful. Sometimes these experiences have been linked to periods of mental ill health and sometimes not. To make sense of this, it is necessary to study my spiritual narrative from my earliest memories (Cardano, 2010; Moran *et al*, 2012). This is helpful to me as an individual, but also can have implications for others in a similar situation (Gockel, 2009; Kogstad *et al*, 2011). Of course, this is anecdotal, but I hope that it will provide ideas for future research.

## My journey

### Experiencing religious well-being

One of my earliest memories is when I was about 5 years old and unable to sleep one night. It seemed to me that God was telling me that I must become a missionary, healing the sick in foreign lands, somewhere where the people had nothing, no medicines, no hospitals. Yes, I said to God, I will do that. I was very happy about it and believed I might be able to really 'make a difference'. I told no one, not even my parents, but I fantasized about it. It is always hard to know how to interpret these kinds of experiences. However, my religious beliefs were certainly sincere and provided me with the sense of meaning and purpose that we would call religious well-being.

I maintain, even after all this time and all that has happened since, that this was a true calling from God. The problem was that I took it too literally, and also used it to help me feel important. We are all 'called by God', but each in our own individual way.

## *Religion replaced by music*

As I grew up, my calling from God faded and my experience of religious well-being declined. I was socially inept and definitely unhappy. The only thing that I lived for was coming top in the exams and trying to play the piano. At that time I did not have much spiritual or religious well-being. Certainly the goal to succeed in every examination does not classify as a spiritual one. It was not even striving for excellence for its own sake.

Then, quite unexpectedly, I started to learn how to play the violin. You could say it was a God-given opportunity and it certainly has transformed my life. Although I already had some skills in playing the piano, this never meant anything as much as my love affair with my violin. My motive was plain to see – I just loved it. I developed a passion for music, realizing it was a far greater thing than something I had to succeed in on my own. I really wanted to play all these wonderful tunes that I heard, written by other people. I really wanted to be involved with other people making music that was much greater than the sum of the individual parts.

I began to listen to a lot of different classical music. The variety, the beauty and the excitement of it fascinated me. Eventually I became good enough to play in an orchestra and I lived for every Saturday afternoon when we rehearsed. Even now I know every note of many of the pieces we played. For me at that time, my music provided me with spiritual well-being, not specifically religious but transcending earthly experiences. Surely this is evidence of the God-given spiritual power of music.

## *Religion returns*

Meanwhile my religious faith was returning, though in a rather unhelpful way. Although I believed in God, I became obsessed with my own sin and inability to do anything about it. When I was 14, I was confirmed, determined to do better and become a Christian 'properly'. I was then influenced by the Christian Union in my school and somehow managed to believe that I needed to be converted all over again. I re-committed myself and naively expected that life would be different. This happened repeatedly and I felt progressively more and more guilty. Why my faith was no longer helpful to me was not clear. Part of it was certainly a flawed idea about what the experience of 'becoming a Christian' actually meant. Perhaps I was expecting that I would feel that Jesus would tangibly fill the gap that friends would have filled if I had any. In addition, at home, I always felt I was not 'good enough', and of course people tend to base their initial image of God on their early life experience. In contrast to my musical experience at the time, my religion was not helping me, and I was certainly not experiencing religious well-being.

## *Continued spiritual well-being through music*

As I reached the sixth form I became obsessed by doing well in my A-level examinations and getting a place at university. In the end I went off to study medicine. I had lost my sense of calling but I was determined that somehow I would make a go of it. What kept me going was my music. I found real joy in playing with other people and making something that seemed to transcend ordinary life. Playing string quartets is still my most favourite occupation. The intimacy of the communication between the four players has a depth to it that is truly spiritual; it goes far beyond anything that could be expressed in words. It gave me something to live for and some contact with other people.

## *Religious ill-being begins*

It was in my second year at university that everything began to unravel. My struggles keeping up with work and my growing social isolation caused me to seek help again in the church. I had been spasmodically attending a church since arriving at university. Now I became obsessed with religion and was convinced that I was neither properly converted nor properly committed. Each week I felt I needed to be evangelized. My constant inability to believe that I was already a Christian had a profound negative impact on me. Despite this I kept on going to the church. Yes, my religion was important to me, and I wanted to find strength, guidance and inspiration from God to help me in my daily struggles, but somehow it was actually causing me problems in itself. I was experiencing religious ill-being.

One day when I was sitting in church I heard what I thought was the voice of the Devil calling me. I was petrified. It was very insistent. I do not know why I thought it was the Devil; it just was, and I just knew. He was threatening to control me and said that I did not belong to Christ. I sat there for a while paralyzed with fright, and finally left the church without speaking to anyone, in a very distressed state. After this, I did not go to the church for a few weeks, but finally the desperation of wanting help led me back there. Unfortunately, the same thing happened and the Devil returned to torment me. At this stage I only had those experiences when I went to church. Eventually I plucked up courage to ask one of the ministers for some help. The next thing that happened was probably the most frightening experience that I have ever had. The priest thought that I was possessed by a demon, and something needed to be done about it. He then performed an exorcism in order to remove the offending Devil.

### Interpretation of religious ill-being

All kinds of questions are raised by this sequence of events. In all cultures and within all religions, peoples' mental state has been associated with disturbances in their religious experiences. Within Christianity this may involve demons or Devils, within a Muslim culture they are known as Jinns, or in India, *bhuts*, and in other cultures as evil spirits. When 'demon possession' is diagnosed by religious leaders, exorcism may be recommended as a suitable treatment. There is anecdotal evidence for the effectiveness of this therapy, but there is much disagreement about whether it is ever curative in the long term (Page, 1989; Wilson, 1989; Rosik, 1997; Stafford, 2005). There is evidence that it can even cause long-term emotional or spiritual damage (Fraser, 1993). Although most Western psychiatry now discounts such treatments, strong belief in them persists among different faith communities.

Considering my own situation at that time, I did indeed think that I had somehow allowed or even encouraged the Devils to enter my life. However, I had never knowingly invited any demon into my life and I had never had any dealings with the occult. I was just a lonely, unhappy, frightened and mixed-up student. It is unlikely that the exorcism was an appropriate treatment for me at that time.

## Coping with religious ill-being

The few weeks after the exorcism were remarkably positive. I felt on a bit of a high, and much more confident with work. I just about managed to attend church and thought I was coping rather better. However, this did not last long. The Devil then returned, bringing what I assumed to be all his pals with him. Again, I had an exorcism, and again they returned. Each time, things became worse than the time before. Every now and again, I was having the same problems when I was not in church. Eventually I became cynical of the exorcism approach and stopped going to church altogether. I came to accept that these Devils talking about me were an inevitable part of my life, and somehow I had to deal with the situation.

## *Persistence of spiritual well-being through music*

Although I could not find comfort in my religion, I still sought solace in my music. Now I cut myself off from other people and just played on my own. My favourite was unaccompanied Bach, the sonatas and partitas. When I could not cope with work I skived off to the hospital chapel and enjoyed the lovely acoustic. I had a secret yearning to play the violin professionally, but I knew how competitive it was, how stressful auditions would be, and how unhappy my parents would be with that decision.

Even though my difficult religious experiences were interfering with my life, I managed to pass my examinations. I never thought that I would give up medicine so I carried on, trying not to look too hard into the future.

## *Spiritual and religious ill-being coincide*

Over the next few years I became more and more isolated and unhappy. I did not darken the door of any church. By now I was doing my clinical course, supposedly learning the practical skills of being a doctor. I found going on to any hospital ward completely terrifying and could not learn anything that way. My solution was to opt out, in other words just not to turn up to ward rounds at all.

My religious difficulties persisted and were actually getting worse. It became too emotionally painful for me to play my violin and I became progressively more nervous, such that I could not even play on my own, with no one else present. My days of finding refuge in music were, for the moment, over.

You may ask, why did I not seek help from anyone? Well, I had tried the church and not found it helpful. I did try at one point to get advice from various doctors, none of whom I managed to trust. Various people put me on various medications, but none of them seemed to help. I have to take responsibility for not having the courage to be open with people and I deeply regret not having done so at that point.

## Crisis on its way

Somehow I managed to pass my finals. Given that I had hardly spent any time on the wards and that I had learnt how to examine a patient out of a book with no practical experience, this was no mean feat. Of course the obvious consequence was that I had now got to work as a doctor without the practical experience that I really needed. And at the same time my experiences were making it very difficult for me to concentrate on anything. I became more and more distracted and less and less competent at my job. My so-called religion had become a nightmare and I started to think that bad things were coming out of my violin when I tried to play.

At this point I think anyone would agree that I had lost my spiritual well-being. I was losing my motivation, I had no sense of who I was or wanted to be and no social contact. I could see no purpose, hope or beauty in life and was gradually giving up the struggle. I also had what I would call a warped spiritual sense that was in itself contributing to my suffering and difficulties. The anguish, despair, self-hate, the conviction that I could only ever hurt people rather than help them and the idea that God was very angry with me, all were the consequences of my spirituality going all wrong, actual spiritual and religious ill-being.

At the end of that year of working as a doctor I was completely incapable of doing the job. I believed that I had actually invited the Devil into my life, that I had committed many unforgivable sins, that I was being suitably punished, and that through me, evil was destroying the whole world. I felt consumed with guilt about letting my parents down and felt so bad about myself that I believed I had a duty to take my own life. In fact there was so much going on in my head that I could not hold a conversation.

## The lowest point
### Experiencing despair

This was the lowest point of my life so far. I attempted to take my own life and in the process, although I cannot remember much about it, I found myself a patient in a psychiatric hospital. Before this time I had not really thought of myself as being mentally unwell; I just knew that I was being tormented. It was all a huge shock for me. I was consumed with guilt and felt very ashamed of having virtually given up on life. I felt dreadful about causing my parents so much distress. The violin had somehow arrived in the hospital and was under my bed in the dormitory, but the very thought of even looking at it was too much.

My exact diagnosis was not established for a very long time. I did not make it easy for the staff to help me as I was practically mute for many months. This was primarily because I could not concentrate on a conversation. On top of that, the staff did not win my trust. They seemed to be impatient and annoyed with me; they suggested that I should have known better as I was a doctor, and they teased me for putting on weight with all the medication they filled me up with. They were probably frustrated because they did not know what to do with me and I was not getting better despite their cocktail of drugs. Telling narratives of any sort was an impossibility, however helpful that might have been.

## *Mental illness or a religious catastrophe?*

The question is, were my religious problems part of a psychiatric illness, were they actual problems with my religion, or were they a bit of both? I had obvious spiritual ill-being, but now I also had a new label – a patient in a psychiatric hospital who had just attempted suicide. This sort of problem requires expert discernment (Hodge, 2004). Basically, if a religious conviction is damaging and coexists with symptoms of recognizable mental illness, then it is likely that the experiences are part of this mental illness. If someone has misconceptions about their faith, this suggests some degree of specifically religious problems. Often people have both problems coexisting. I believe that most mental illness has a spiritual dimension, just as it has biological, social and psychological dimensions (Clarke, 2009).

Looking back on it, I almost certainly had a mental illness, but with a big spiritual/religious dimension. Since I had never dabbled in the occult or anything like it, it was unlikely to have been solely a religious problem. It had not responded to the obvious 'religious' solutions of exorcism and repeated religious conversion, and my experiences could be interpreted as hallucinations and delusions within a mental illness. However, I did have specifically religious problems in that I undoubtedly had a skewed image of God and many misunderstandings about the Christian faith and expectations of life. The medication that I was given did not by any means 'cure' my problems. I believe I actually needed the right sort of help with my religion as well as treatment for mental illness, and that neither one nor the other would suffice.

## *A purposeless existence*

I stayed on that hospital ward for the best part of 5 years and at the end of that time I was not that much better than I had been when I had been admitted. All this time I had not confided in the staff on the ward about my religious experiences because I was ashamed, frightened and I could not bring myself to trust sufficiently. I found my stubborn streak and eventually discharged myself, finding a very small bedsit to rent. When it became obvious that I was not coping on my own I went back to live with my parents. I had nothing to do, no job, no friends, and nowhere of my own to go. I am very grateful that my parents took me in at this point, even though it was not an ideal situation. The only other option seemed to be some sort of institution.

## New beginnings

Shortly after moving the inevitable happened and I found myself back in hospital. As I had now moved to a different area, I was under the care of a different mental health team. This time I managed to confide in the staff team and told them something about my religious experiences. They realized that I found sharing these things very difficult and they were very patient with me. One psychiatrist in particular somehow won my trust and he became my consultant for many years. He showed interest in me as a person rather than just a walking mental health problem. He looked after my spiritual well-being in the broadest sense. This included not only trying to understand what was important to me in life, but also encouraging me in many practical ways. The first thing he did for me was to get me playing my violin again. Even though this was a long and difficult journey, it did provide me with an invaluable source of spiritual well-being. I had not played at all for 7 years, so getting back my skill was a huge challenge. However, it gave me something to focus on, which was just what I needed at the time.

## Renewed spiritual well-being at last

It took years for me to find something really satisfying to do. When I did, it was my consultant who facilitated this. All my years spent on a hospital ward inspired me to want to help others who were in this situation. I thought of people with advanced dementia, stuck in a hospital or care home, with little to connect them to life. I knew they had very little occupational therapy or entertainment. I had the idea that I could take my violin and entertain them myself. My consultant put me in touch with the manager of a ward that he considered might be suitable. Of course, I was hideously nervous. Somehow I managed it and this activity occupied me for the following 10 years. I still do it once a week to this day. Over the years I have recorded my own backing tracks and invented many different programmes of things to play. Often people join in singing, even dancing to the music. This has provided me with purpose in life, true spiritual well-being, and even joy on occasions. It has sustained me even when my religious difficulties have troubled me most.

Another source of spiritual well-being for me has been playing in a local amateur orchestra, which I joined about 15 years ago. It has given me the opportunity to recapture the inspiration of playing in many great pieces of music over the years. Although it has often been a source of much stress, I have kept going with it, and it is getting easier.

## Telling my religious narrative

Throughout all this time, I had frequent relapses when things got the better of me. Over months and years I developed more trust in my consultant. He seemed to believe in me and genuinely care about me. He showed this even in small practical ways, for example, finding me some lunch one day when I was in a bad way. This trust enabled me to share my religious experiences in more detail with him. This was the first time that I had ever shared my religious narrative with anyone. He validated my experiences patiently and compassionately, understanding their implications for the way I feel and think about my life. He realized that I did indeed need some help with my religious beliefs and experiences, and being an atheist himself, he was not the right person to provide this. He arranged for me to see a mental health chaplain. She was crucial for my recovery.

With her I explored my religious journey from when I was very young, sharing my religious narrative in a way I had never done before. The result was that I began to understand why I had developed religious problems. I learnt things that might be seen as obvious, such as that God must be more important and powerful than my Devils, and that being Devils, they most likely lie to me anyway. I could look back on my repeated conversions, my exorcisms, and my failure to fulfil my childhood calling, as all contributing to my excessive guilt. However, despite all this, I have never totally discounted the validity of my experiences as originating from my own sin and inner evil. Mostly, I can sit well balanced on the fence, as it were, and sometimes I even manage to reject my religious experiences totally. Sometimes, I topple over onto the other side.

I try not to think about it too much.

I talked at length with the chaplain about attending a church and perhaps becoming part of a faith community. One day, I was passing a church in the city centre where I live and a service was in progress. I was inspired to go in. This was the first time I had been to a church service for quite a few years and I did not know how I would react. Of course it was traumatic. However, I immediately felt that this was a tolerant place and that the people there might accept even me. The sermon was about divorced Christians and gay Christians and how they can all be part of God's community. Although I cried throughout the service, and spoke to no one, I left feeling that I might go back one day.

## *Religious well-being at last*

There followed a time of hope. In fact, the hope I felt at that point was greater than anything I had felt since that calling when I was 5 years old. I began to attend that church regularly. I have never found it easy to 'worship' God with prayer or singing worship songs, and never feel the deep ecstasy that many people find when they praise and worship. At first, I felt guilty about this. However, I started to realise that perhaps my playing is my way of worshipping. I have met many lovely people at that church, and now I actually have friends there. I feel accepted in whatever state I am when I turn up there. I feel supported by this faith community.

## Spiritual and religious well-being coincide

My consultant came up with yet more suggestions. I always had a research interest and he put me in touch with a colleague from the local university who was passionate in getting service users involved in research. I am now involved in some research, which is giving me a huge sense of purpose that I have never had before and has improved my spiritual well-being even further. This research is about spirituality in mental illness and how this can be nurtured. This is the basis of what we call 'spiritual care' (Culliford, 2007; Galanter *et al*, 2011). I was, of course, inspired to get involved with this because of my own experiences.

The first project was with the production of the *Handbook of Spiritual Care in Mental Illness*, which outlines the theory behind spiritual care and how it is best achieved (it is available at www.bsmhft.nhs.uk/service-user-and-carer/service-user-information/spiritual-care). This involves service users telling their spiritual narratives. The process begins with a routine spiritual assessment or brief spiritual narrative, in which a brief description of the person's spiritual life from childhood to the present day is noted (Puchalski, 2006). A spiritual care plan is made on the basis of this, incorporating the person's wishes (Galanter *et al*, 2011). This often involves further exploration of their spiritual experiences with a person of their choice, including perhaps a more detailed narrative.

My aim is to contribute to the evaluation of spiritual care, which I believe is crucial for recovery for many service users. At present I am attempting to validate an appropriate assessment tool with which we might be able to do this.

My other sources of spiritual and religious well-being have persisted and actually grown. I still play my violin for other service users, play in the orchestra and attend church. I have friends. I have a sense of meaning and hope for the future. But above all, I have a sense of religious well-being. I am hugely grateful to God that He has helped me to reach this point. I dare to say that I believe that God somehow forgives me, cares about me, loves even me and has a purpose for my life in the time I have left on this earth. I am trying to trust His guidance in my life. Of course, I fall down frequently and experience relapses every now and then, but I have more insight now. I know when to seek help, and what helps and what does not.

## What spirituality has come to mean to me

### What do I mean by spiritual?

For me, spirituality is whatever gives any individual person meaning, purpose and hope to keep going in life (Barber *et al*, 2012) and does not have to include a formal religion. In common with most people with mental health problems (Mohr *et al*, 2007; Reinart & Koenig, 2013), my spirituality is very important to me and has been shaped by my life experiences over the years. My spiritual life has two major facets, the first concerning my Christian religion and the second concerning my love of music, which I think of as spiritual in a broader sense (Wlodarczyk, 2007). My religious faith is the more obviously spiritual source of inspiration. However, I have often relied on music as a spiritual outlet when my religion has been problematic for me.

### Spiritual well-being and spiritual ill-being

It is generally assumed that our spirituality and/or our religion has positive and helpful consequences for us, and that it promotes our well-being. I use the term 'spiritual well-being' to describe this phenomenon (Ivstan *et al*, 2013) and I distinguish between 'spiritual' and 'religious' well-being depending on whether or not a formal religion is involved.

Sometimes, however, our spirituality goes wrong. A considerable subset of people with mental health problems actually struggle with their spirituality, especially when this involves religious issues, and it becomes a problem in itself (Mohr & Huguelet, 2004; McConnell *et al*, 2006; Mohr *et al*, 2006, 2011). I have frequently had this experience. I choose to call this phenomenon religious or spiritual 'ill-being'.

## In conclusion

So I come round full circle. My childhood dream was based on religious well-being and a calling from God. I discovered the joy of music and that has sustained me through many problems. I then went through a huge loss including experiencing religious ill-being, and then eventually spiritual ill-being when nothing seemed to help me. My life fell apart and there were wasted years. But gradually my music returned to give me a new sense of purpose and spiritual well-being in a way that I had least expected. I have now become involved in a research project. Finally, I have a sense of God's purpose again and have found renewed religious well-being.

Many people have helped me on this journey. My consultant provided acceptance, understanding, encouragement, crucial support and insight. The chaplain has helped me to sort out what I really believe and why. And there have been other people, psychiatric nurses, a psychologist, people I have met through my work and, more recently, people from the church. You might ask, how have these people actually helped me? Most of all, they have enabled and encouraged me to tell my spiritual narrative, walked through it with me, and helped me make sense of it and learn from my experiences. Spiritual and religious well-being continue to be the most important things in my life. I truly believe that this is the same for many other struggling service users. Telling your spiritual narrative is often therapeutic in itself and I believe that this opportunity should be available for all as part of routine spiritual care.

# References

Barber, J.M., Parkes, M., Parsons, H., *et al* (2012) Importance of spiritual well-being in the assessment of recovery, the Service user Recovery Evaluation Scale (SeRvE). *Psychiatrist*, 36, 444–50.

Cardano, M. (2010) Mental distress: strategies of sense making. *Health*, 14, 253–73.

Clarke, J. (2009) A critical view of how nursing has defined spirituality. *Journal of Clinical Nursing*, 18, 1666–73.

Culliford, L. (2007) Taking a spiritual history. *Advances in Psychiatric Treatment*, 13, 212–19.

Fraser, G.A. (1993) Exorcism rituals: effects on multiple personality disorder patients. *Dissociation*, 6, 239–44.

Galanter, M., Dermatis, H., Talbot, N., *et al* (2011) Introducing spirituality into psychiatric care. *Journal of Religion and Health*, 50, 81–91.

Gockel, A. (2009) Spirituality and the process of healing: a narrative study. *International Journal for the Psychology of Religion*, 19, 217–30.

Hodge, D.R. (2004) Spirituality and people with mental illness: developing spiritual competency in assessment and intervention. *Families in Society*, 85, 36–45.

Ivstan, I., Chan, C.P.L. & Gardner, H.E. (2013) Linking religion and spirituality with psychological well-being: examining self-actualisation, meaning in life and personal growth initiative. *Journal of Religion and Health*, 52, 915–29.

Kogstad, R.E., Ekeland, T.-J. & Hummelroll, J.K. (2011) In defence of a humanistic approach to mental health care: recovery process investigated with the help of client's narratives on turning points and process of gradual change. *Journal of Psychiatric and Mental Health Nursing*, 18, 479–86.

McConnell, K.M., Pargament, K.I., Ellison, C.G., *et al* (2006) Examining the links between spiritual struggles and symptoms of psychopathology in a national sample. *Journal of Clinical Psychology*, 62, 1469–84.

Mohr, S. & Huguelet, P. (2004) The relationship between schizophrenia and religion and its implications for care. *Swiss Medical Weekly*, 134, 369–76.

Mohr, S., Brandt, P.-Y., Borras, L., *et al* (2006) Towards an integration of spirituality and religiousness into the psychological dimension of schizophrenia. *American Journal of Psychiatry*, 163, 1952–9.

Mohr, S., Gillieron, C., Borras, L., *et al* (2007) The assessment of spirituality and religiousness in schizophrenia. *Journal of Nervous and Mental Disease*, 195, 247–53.

Mohr, S., Perroud, N., Gillieron, C., *et al* (2011) Spirituality and religiousness as predictive factors of outcome in schizophrenia and schizo-affective disorders. *Psychiatry*, 186, 177–82.

Moran, G.S., Russinova, Z., Gidugu, V., *et al* (2012) Benefits and mechanisms of recovery among peer providers with psychiatric illness. *Qualitative Health Research*, 22, 304–19.

Page, S.H.T. (1989) The role of exorcism in clinical practice and pastoral care. *Journal of Psychology and Theology,* **17,** 121–31.

Puchalski, C.M. (2006) Spiritual assessment in clinical practice. *Psychiatric Annals,* **36,** 150–5.

Reinart, K.G. & Koenig, H.G. (2013) Re-examining definitions in spirituality in nursing research. *Journal of Advanced Nursing,* **69,** 2622–34.

Rogers, S.A., Malony, H.N., Coleman, E.M., *et al* (2002) Changes in attitudes towards religion among those with mental illness. *Journal of Religion and Health,* **41,** 167–79.

Rosik, C.H. (1997) When discernment fails: the case for outcome studies on exorcism. *Journal of Psychology and Theology,* **25,** 354–63.

Stafford, B. (2005) The growing evidence for 'demonic possession': What psychiatry's response should be? *Journal of Religion and Health,* **44,** 13–31.

Wilson, W.P. (1989) Demon possession and exorcism: A Reaction to Page. *Journal of Psychology and Theology,* **17,** 135–9.

Wlodarczyk, N. (2007) The effect of music therapy on the spirituality of persons in an in-patient hospice unit as measured by self report. *Journal of Music Therapy,* **44,** 113–23.

CHAPTER 11

# God's story revealed in the human story

Beaumont Stevenson

How does the existence of God, or a higher power, make itself apparent in our own story as human beings? The evidence of divine presence would have to be in a form that we human beings could recognize. While we have empirical ways of evaluating facts, the presence of God would require us to acknowledge a different dimension to our own. It would have to include relationship on a higher scale, evidence of care and involvement, and perhaps also stories from our history demonstrating the continuity of this greater relationship with humankind.

The human intellect, being grounded in time and space can never comprehend God's story in full. Yet the human heart takes us further; through its actions we see the Divine at work. In this chapter I would like to explore how that divine presence may be felt, experienced and recognized in the narratives of individuals' lives and in their communities. In particular, I hope to show how spiritual narrative can help people with mental health problems connect with this greater being and purpose.

I begin with a story about the desert, and how this desert experience was reflected in the lives of the 'desert experience' that individuals go through in a psychiatric hospital. I will then look at how different levels of reality – especially the spiritual one – can be accessed through metaphor or stories. Conclusions will then be drawn from these experiences and examples.

## Spirituality: belonging to more than myself

An important realisation came to me as a young man when I was attending a series of lectures given by the French theologian Samuel Terrien, at the Episcopal Theological School in Cambridge, Massachusetts, in 1963. Terrien said something that changed my life – that the great religions of Judaism, Christianity and Islam were all born in the desert. He added that if you are serious about your spiritual search for meaning, you must go to the desert yourself; only there will you truly be able to understand. In the desert, you are aware that you can die and no one would ever find you.

You see the narrow edge between yourself and survival, and the distant stars are brighter. Somehow, in that place, you are aware that you are not alone and there is a presence with you of which ordinarily you might not be aware because of the distractions of civilization.

Terrien then shared some of his own experiences of the desert. He attached himself to a caravan travelling across the desert and occasionally they would encounter another caravan. They might discover that the members of another passing caravan were relations of theirs, many times removed. They would then camp for several days together, while each group shared the story of their branch of their common family history, filling in the gaps in their history about which the other relatives would not know. Sometimes these story-sharing times would take several days; the oral tradition meant that everyone knew their family story without it being written down. Hearing the story once meant that it would be remembered by all.

In this sense, perhaps it can be said that 'his-story' becomes attached to 'my-our story' and *vice versa*, adding a greater depth of meaning to 'my-our identity' and helping to define my-our particular place in an all-encompassing story. It is probably no coincidence that *The Canterbury Tales* were told between individuals who were on a pilgrimage – stories that connect the spiritual journey with a meaningful narrative. Similarly with Alcoholics Anonymous, where the healing process encourages people to tell their particular story to others and in doing so, later to connect this story with the discovery of a higher power. Likewise, there is a connection between group psychotherapy and spirituality. Irving Yalom reports that hearing other people's stories promotes the feeling of universality among group members, in that each realizes there is a connection between themselves and their experience, and the human race as seen in other individuals' stories (Yalom, 1975: pp. 7–9).

## Experiencing the self not as part but whole

Michael Wilson (1988) describes the difference between illness and disease as follows: disease is what is wrong, but illness is when the part takes over the whole. He gives the example of a group of adolescents who stole a car and were joyriding around the city. They had a crash. The disease was handled when they were taken to casualty and their injuries sewn up; the illness, however, was when their parents were contacted and it transpired that none of the parents knew or cared where their children were. Wilson quotes Shattuck in saying, rather colourfully, 'sometimes it is more important to know what kind of fella has a germ than what kind of germ is in the fella' (p. 36).

When our illness threatens to become our identity, how do we find the wider perspective and see the whole rather than the part?

This is illustrated by a story told by the psychiatrist Viktor Frankl (1984), who encountered a woman cleaner in the hospital in Vienna where he worked:

> The woman told Frankl that because she was old and ill and could not clean and scrub floors anymore, she was useless. In reply, he asked her to tell him her story. She related that she and her husband had raised four children, two of whom were teachers, one was in business and one was a doctor. During the war the rest of her family had been killed. Frankl asked her to concentrate on one of her sons, the one who was the doctor, and asked how many people he might have seen in one afternoon:
>
> 'Ten' she said.
>
> 'What if he had cured two of those patients on that particular afternoon by successfully treating their illness; where would the result of that one afternoon be at the moment?' Frankl replied.
>
> She said that they would have been able to return to their families, possibly have more children and might have been able to contribute to others through their lives and work.
>
> 'Where would that afternoon be felt?' asked Frankl.
>
> 'All over the world', she answered.
>
> Frankl pointed out that this had been just one afternoon in one of her children's lives and all that was made possible because she scrubbed floors. He then asked her if she still thoguht she was useless. She replied that she was very valuable and had even influenced the lives of people who never knew of her existence. She could now see a connection between her life and history in a new way. Her identity had changed from that of her illness, which made her 'useless', to the discovery of significance and meaning.

## Spiritual narratives in a mental health community

Let us explore the mechanism of how special our particular history is in influencing others, sometimes by our very limitations rather than our skills.

As chaplain of a psychiatric hospital, I had not worked there for long before I realized that because many patients had a patch over their eye of reason, it enabled them to see more clearly things to which more reasonable people were blind; like the desert experience, without the glare of logic distant stars were brighter. I observed that these people were often more aware of the spiritual dimension, reminiscent of the biblical prophets. Not being burdened with reason, they were clearer about a higher dimension.

> One day in the chapel of the psychiatric hospital, I was administering Holy Communion. When I came to a lady kneeling at the communion rail, she screamed and shouted: 'I am not worthy' and collapsed over the rail sobbing.
>
> Quick as a flash, the lady kneeling next to her said: 'In that case, have a Polo mint, my dear' and offered her one. The distressed lady looked somewhat surprised.
>
> As chaplain, I added, 'You may either have the sacrament or a Polo mint; whatever you feel you need just now.'
>
> She replied that she would have to think about it. She thought and we waited; we waited and she thought some more. Finally came the reply.

'I think I'll stick with the Polo mint', she said. She took one and I gave her a blessing.

Next week she was back. Coming to the rail, she held her thumb in the air and shouted 'Worthy this week, Father!' Everyone applauded.

At the end of the service, I said to the congregation that I wanted them to be aware that a minor miracle might have happened. I said that when we are feeling poorly we cannot have solid food, so we have to have broth instead. Having received the broth of the Polo mint last week, given her through the priesthood of a fellow patient, she was enabled to have the more solid spiritual meal this week. I asked them to reflect on how they might have been priests to one another during the past week and how others might have been a priest to them. They thought about it and many nodded their heads in agreement.

On another occasion, my colleague was celebrating the Eucharist. He told the congregation that ordinarily they would be asked to pray for whatever they liked during the service during the prayers, but that this week he was going to ask them to have a discussion among themselves and all decide together as a group on just one thing to pray for. Puzzled a bit, they agreed and after a somewhat lengthy discussion their spokesperson said: 'We have decided we want someone to make us laugh as it is so depressing being in a place like this.'

The chaplain replied that maybe Beau might be able to make them laugh, but that he himself did not feel able to as he was more serious; but their prayer would be offered as requested.

Then, just when the priest was saying the prayer of consecration, at the 'holiest moment' of the prayer a member of the congregation said aloud:

> 'Hey, have you heard the news that scientists have just discovered that diarrhoea is inherited?'
>
> 'No!' said several people, 'we didn't.'
>
> 'Yes,' replied the speaker 'it runs in your jeans.'

Everyone collapsed with laughter, including the priest who was so convulsed that he had to stop for breath before he could continue.

During a subsequent supervision session, the priest and I explored what had happened. Several things came up: first that the word 'someone' seemed to refer to someone in authority who would have the 'cure' to being in a depressive place – perhaps a doctor, nurse, or the officiating chaplain. The priest had fallen into this assumption by suggesting that another someone (Beau) might be that particular laughter expert. The corporate surprise was that a fellow sufferer did it, and at precisely the holiest part of the service, where Christ became 'earthed in bread' – and so it became a healing moment where the participants were able to connect to universality in shared laughter.

This also reflected a style that Jesus often used, namely, metaphors open to ambiguity, in this case with a pun about scientists finding out how much mental illness runs in our genes.

## Ways in which spiritual narratives heal

### Metaphor

*Meta* in Greek means 'beyond' and *phor* comes from *phoros* or 'carrying'. A metaphor speaks about one thing in terms suggestive of another (Soskice, 1985). Metaphor provides meaning through a more overarching context than the current predicament in which we find ourselves, thereby furnishing a more inclusive map, a verbal image, which can bring a wider and sometimes more surprising way of seeing where we are stuck. Metaphor resists analysis because it bypasses logic, providing an unexpected new dimension of meaning.

The power of metaphor in narrative is that it expands the possibilities for meaning, and especially for spiritual or religious meaning. Indeed, theology and religion rely extensively on metaphor, as ordinary language is far too limited as a means of talking about God. Jesus, for example, appears to use metaphor in order to bring a wider perspective to narrow religious views of dos and don'ts.

### Symbol

Within the narrative lie symbols, which stand for something larger than themselves. The word means 'to throw things together'. It gathers something complicated and puts it in one place.

Interestingly, the opposite of symbol is *diabol*, a word commonly associated with the Devil, meaning 'to break things apart into constituent elements' – the opposite of unity. The Devil tests Jesus before his ministry begins by putting smaller truths before him: 'Look after yourself by turning stones into bread', 'Throw yourself off the temple so the populace will say: "Wow, how did he do that!"'

Imagine yourself seated across a candle-lit table from the person you love the most. Taking your beloved's hand, you look deeply in their eyes and say 'Could you consider entering into a formal contract where we legally cohabit and perhaps mix genes producing subsequent progeny?' This is an example of *diabol*, factually accurate but entirely missing the level to which symbolic language might transport the couple.

In contrast, the symbol fuses disparate parts into a whole. It makes us aware of the common ground that supports us and on which we base our lives. Accordingly, it lends itself to the Sacred.

### Living in the eternal now

In the Old Testament story of Moses meeting God in the burning bush that is not consumed (Exodus 3) God asks Moses to take off his shoes because he is standing on holy ground. Moses asks God what his name is. This is an impossible question because a name defines one thing from another and that which is infinite is therefore beyond definition. God answers that he is

'I AM' – the present tense of the verb 'to be'. God is therefore in the 'now' of things and it means that wherever we stand in the present moment we face the possibility of encountering eternal being. It is usually difficult to sustain being fully in the 'now'; our tendency is rather to fixate on our past and worry in anticipation of the future.

Patrick Carroll, in his book *Where God May Be Found* (1994) puts the story of Moses' encounter with God in a delightful form. God says:

> 'Take off your shoes, Moses, you are standing on Holy Ground.' And Moses replies (it is not in the book, but he must have said it) 'But this is the ground I always stand on.' And the bush replies 'Right!'
>
> We stand on holy ground all the time. Moses talked to God out in the fields where he watches his flocks, not in the temple. Go on with the story.
>
> Imagine Moses coming home that night and saying to his wife,
>
> 'Honey, we're going back to Egypt! We're going to set our people free.' And she says, 'We can't go back there. You're wanted for murder.'
>
> Moses says, 'I know, but we have to go.'
>
> 'Who told you?'
>
> 'A bush!'
>
> 'Right.' (pp. 10–11)

So the question arises, how do we change our overall perspective, especially if it becomes entrenched in a limited way or becomes punitive?

## *'Writing' a new story*

We all construct our identities around a personal narrative that helps us make sense of the world and how we experience it. Mostly it fits in with how others see us and then we are deemed to be of sound mind. When the 'fit' is discordant, suffering usually arises. If we can, we may try to challenge compassionately the narrative of the self that is causing distress.

'I'm glad I'm not in your head!', a chaplain colleague of mine said to a woman whose religious views were basically not only punitive but retaliatory. She had been feeling punished inside, and therefore punished outwardly. My colleague asked if she read the same Bible he did, because her religious 'take' on it left out the joyous, the forgiving and the loving. God's voice to her was the voice of criticism, judgement and competition rather than compassion. If our narrative inner voice becomes negative, how might we change it?

Someone I saw once had a similar negative internal voice and I suggested that she take on a guest narrator for a week. She could not think of one, so I suggested Dawn French as 'vicar of Dibley'. She came back the following week and reported that she laughed at everything for 2 days but then it became tiresome, so she switched to her grandmother's voice as narrator which was kind but practical and more supportive. It was such a relief that she decided to make that voice her consistent one.

In an eating disorder unit, adolescent girls would often idealize their fathers (who were not ideal) and instead take the negativity of their fathers into themselves. If the father idealization was coloured by religious perfectionism, this could result in a religious guilt. When this happened in female patients I would get a telephone call from the unit to 'come and do my thing' as chaplain. Changing out of my usual casual attire, I would put on a formal black suit with clerical collar and black polished shoes. I held a leather-bound Bible with gold gilt under my arm, arriving at the unit as a fully accredited conservative churchman. The conversation would go something like this: we would agree on basic Christian doctrine, then I would add: 'Jesus was, of course, without sin, except on one particular occasion where he almost sinned, but was saved from doing so by a gentile woman'. Turning to Mark 7: 24–30 in my Bible, I would share the encounter of Jesus the Jew with a gentile woman. The woman's daughter was ill and she shouted for his attention. First the disciples tried to send her away, but then Jesus himself told her that it was not right to take the children's bread (children being Jews) and throw it to the dogs (non-Jewish gentiles). In the Greek of the New Testament he calls her a female dog (*kunaria*), which means 'bitch'. The woman was not having any of his Jewish prejudice and retorted: 'Bitches have their rights too – we can eat the scraps from the master (*race's*) table. Do you have any scraps to throw me?' Jesus, shocked and perhaps a little surprised by her outburst, heals her 'for her saying', not for her faith as he usually does. In short, she showed up his prejudice and in doing so may have cured Jesus of a prejudice against non-Jews. The implied message is that it is possible for a woman to stand up against arrogant father figures, even one's own. This discussion would quite often open the door to the individual getting better and many changed dramatically after the visit.

## *Reframing the delusional*

Often, delusional ideas are seen as so preposterous or bizarre that they effectively isolate the person, or invoke kindly condescension from the mental health professional, who is hoping that medication will take effect. Sometimes we are afraid to engage with the delusion in case it makes matters worse. But there are times when it is worth taking the chance of having a serious conversation – one that is only possible if 'reality' is temporarily suspended.

> I was talking with a patient in the hospital when he suddenly banged the table and shouted: 'Unless you say that I am Jesus Christ, I will leave this room immediately.'
> 
> Matching the tone of voice, I too banged the table and replied: 'Right! And I'm Moses.'
> 
> 'No, you're not; you're Beau!'
> 
> I continued: 'I have listened to your story, so now you listen to mine: it was bitch, bitch, bitch all across the desert. Give them manna, they want fowl, give them fowl, they want water. There's just no pleasing some folks. I go up to the

mountain top with God for the Ten Commandments, and they build a golden calf. God is angry and wants to wipe out the lot, and I have to use my psychiatric nursing skills to talk him down, implying that if he wipes them out he will lose street cred with the Egyptians by saving them – only to wipe them out himself. After that I was looking forward to retirement. I asked God if I could have a nice place in the Promised Land, perhaps with palm trees and a swimming pool.

God replies: 'No Moses; you die!'

'Why, haven't I served you well?'

'Very well, but we can't have two leaders in the Promised Land; we have Joshua, who is a general, and your presence would undermine his authority. You can peek at the Promised Land though, from a tall hill.'

'Thanks a puddle, God. So what is the retirement policy for Messiahs these days?' I ask.

Long silence.

'That's it; I resign as Messiah; I didn't read the fine print; I'm going back to me again'.

Our conversation then returned to a more normal one. The storytelling had broken through the religious delusion and humanity was restored.

## *Transforming I-it into I-Thou*

Bible stories such as the parable of the Good Samaritan (Luke 10: 25–37) have a timeless relevance to the human condition. Here is an up-to-date version of this from one of my discovered gurus at the hospital, who fits the bill as a neighbour and who, by the way she discovered her own neighbour, helped me change my perspective in a surprising way.

> I was late for an appointment and a bit stressed. Driving into the hospital car park, all the places were filled except for one – taken by a lady whom I knew, who was in earnest discussion with a lamp post. Not wishing to interrupt what might have been an important discussion (and a little annoyed too), I kept the car running until she eventually finished her conversation. After I had parked, I approached and asked her: 'What's up?'
>
> She replied that she had been living in the hospital for many years and that she had no living relations. Then she said she met someone in the same boat as herself, who also had no relatives. They talked. The question that came up was what they had each most missed by not having relatives, and the answer was that they never received any gifts. So they decided together to do something about it: from Monday to Wednesday, she said, 'I would go to the shop and buy her cigarettes, chocolate and a surprise; from Thursday to Saturday, the other lady did the same for me, so that every day a gift was given or received. Then she added, 'Yesterday my friend died unexpectedly'.
>
> I felt tearful myself then; after a while I told her that I was sorry about her friend's death, but I felt that she and her friend were not far from the kingdom of God because they had discovered in essence what life was about; that we exist through the care and generosity of others. I thanked her for the gift she had given me with her story, and it did not really seem to matter much that I was late for my appointment, as I had been given a gift. She had 'reached' me with her story and in return, I had offered her my story – that she was closer to heaven on Earth than she perhaps knew. As Martin Buber (1958) has shown,

the 'I-Thou' narrative in which we are engaged brings us into the presence of the Divine, for which no amount of talking with a lamp post can substitute.

## *Finding a place for suffering*

Mental distress has a way of blinding us to the bigger picture in which, paradoxically, opposites live together in the same event. Jesus uses this in the Beatitudes by putting opposites next to one another, to reveal how the positive and negative often come from the same event.

Blessed means 'happy' or 'fulfilled'. Jesus says 'Happy are you who mourn for you will find comfort' (literally, 'to be found with strengths you did not know you had'). 'Happy are you when people abuse you and persecute you and speak all kinds of calumny against you on my account; [...] This is how they persecuted the prophets before you' (*The Jerusalem Bible*, London, 1966: Matthew 5: 11–12). Perhaps there is a parallel here: that if you are in public life and no one ever disagrees with you, you probably are not doing your job properly. Speaking the truth usually causes flak.

For every crisis or difficulty there is an attendant benefit, which is a valuable side-effect. Opposites arise together. Take, for example, the tragic sinking of the Titanic; although it was in itself a terrible disaster, it resulted in badly needed international sea safety regulations which have subsequently saved countless thousands of lives. Crucifixion is a horrific way to die; yet in the Christian tradition, the crucifix becomes a symbol adorned with gold and jewels, and proclaims the good news that there is life after death.

## Seeking the universal in the personal

Peter Reason (2013) takes the view that storytelling can bring about change by responding to an event that someone describes not with analysis but with another story. What emerges is a saga or a myth, which reveals an eternal meaning discerned within ordinary happenings. I have used a similar approach in training clergy to think theologically, and with parishes that seemed to have clouded over their spiritual perspective by descending into warring subgroups around particular contentious issues. The challenge is always how to re-establish the spiritual perspective, which has been lost in the infighting. The process is to gather the group together to share any story that any individual would like. It does not have to be profound (one person described getting a parking ticket). The group does not respond with logic or ordinary exploration of feelings but by drawing pictures, writing poems or telling stories from classical or biblical history. Here is an example of a story that I told and the response someone else gave:

> When I was about 9 years old, I went with my family on vacation to a lake in Northern Michigan, which was near the Great Lakes. My father asked my older brother and myself if we would like to go out in a large boat for some

deep-sea fishing. He said that we would have to get up at 4 am and would be out for most of the day. My brother and I were overjoyed and readily agreed.

We did get up the next morning and went out in the boat, complete with anchored chairs and long fishing poles. We fished without success until the sun was high and it was getting quite hot. Then suddenly my fishing line responded and bent double – excitement all round. The captain and my father both estimated that it was probably a large sturgeon. My older brother was green with envy, which suited me just fine. I told my father that it was too big for me to handle; would he take over the fishing rod? He said no, that it was my fish to either bring in or to lose. However, he said that he would hold me while I held the fishing rod. As I sat on his lap, the struggle went on and on. Then the captain said that something was not quite right. It transpired I had wrapped my fishing line around the boat's propeller! Embarrassed silence from the adult experts as we headed for shore, my father having to pay the captain extra to take his boat out of the water to move the line from the propeller. I wasn't particularly unhappy as I didn't particularly want to have to kill a fish. That was my story.

Then another member of the group followed with this story:

Once upon a time the elder of a tribe took a young boy out in a boat to fish in the waters of a great lake where there were reported to be huge creatures in the Deep. If anyone could catch one of these mythical creatures, they would be given a place of honour in the tribe. All day long they fished in that magical lake. Then it struck! A catch. Was this the great monster which eluded others and which would guarantee the boy's fame? No. It transpired that the boy had caught the boat which contained them instead. Going back to shore, everyone was disappointed except the boy, because he realized that in making the catch as he did, he had discovered something important. He had discovered what he was to do with the rest of his life, which was to enable people to cast into the deep for perhaps the biggest catch of all – to catch their own true self. He had discovered what was to be his life's work.

Needless to say, I was very moved at the insight this re-telling of my story gave through elevating, by means of metaphor and symbol, my personal story into a myth for humanity.

# Walking alongside the other

People with mental illness who are searching to make sense of, and to overcome, their suffering, are often missing something crucial. When in distress, it can be hard for a person to see what higher purpose there may be behind their life story. Finding and then living this higher purpose has been described as vocation – what our uniqueness powerfully calls us to do at this place and at this time. We can look, for instance, at Winston Churchill and see the events of his life leading up to what his unique role was to be during the Second World War. In the pilgrimage, for that is what I think it really is, the storyteller's art, honed in desert experiences, reveals something eternal and ultimate that is lying hidden within the ordinary details of a person's life. My feeling is that with some patients this is expressed in the psychotic (concrete) use of otherwise symbolic language. It might perhaps be a request to be heard and to be understood on this more profound level.

Sometimes there is a shamanic dimension contained within the madness. The shaman becomes 'mad' by opening the self to a different dimension on behalf of the community in which he or she lives. It is to make a journey to another world in order to divine things on a deeper level. The shamanic role also appears in disguise in family therapy. For example, the illness of a particular family member does not come out in the most disturbed member, but often in the weakest member. A distressed child's communication is shamanic in that it reveals what is dysfunctional in another family member. Jesus' death revealed the conflicts within the religions of his time (and ever since), in a way that everyone could see. These days we could put as much on a T-shirt; it might say: 'My madness is us!'

This is vital to the work of both therapist and priest. We try to get alongside someone else's suffering and feel as it must feel for them, not only out of empathy but also to discover a deeper sense of what is going on within the person and the society in which they live. It is exhausting and we feel their turmoil in ourselves if we have the courage (with the help of others) to launder our feelings into insight.

## Small gestures can make a big difference

Soon after my ordination, and in search of my own desert experience, I asked about being assigned to work abroad, and was sent to Zambia. The job entailed helping individuals discuss how they might work together after the country has gained independence, as well as doing some teaching. There was petrol rationing and difficulty with violence at times. While I was visiting the Northern Province I was teaching a class and leading a discussion through an interpreter in a thatched round hovel with an open window. I felt a sharp sting on my hand and looking down saw tsetse fly had just bitten me. Calling the interpreter over, I asked 'Is this a tsetse fly?'

He said that it was and laughed and nodded. He said that there was nothing to worry about. He said if it was not carrying African sleeping sickness, I would be fine; if it was, then I would see the Lord Jesus very soon – so, obviously, nothing at all to worry about! I was not entirely convinced and said that in America it was common when bitten by something nasty to suck the blood out and spit it out, which is what I intended to do. This part of my conversation was not translated. I therefore continued to teach while standing next to an open window and sucking at my wound and spitting it out through the window.

Months later, I was sitting on the veranda at Bishop's House in Lusaka and one of the other priests who had just come back from Northern Province reported that he had encountered something very strange, for every school and church he visited seemed to have a strange custom that he had never seen before. People kissed their hand and spat through the window as they were teaching. He said that it must have been a very ancient custom as everyone seemed to be doing it across the entire region. Embarrassed, I hid behind the paper I was reading.

Before leaving Zambia, when I happened to ask a friend what African name I had been given during my tour of duty, he replied without hesitation 'Batata Malishipa Panse'.

'What did it mean?' I asked.

'Priest who spits through the window', came the reply.

So there it is – my fear of falling ill had, I would like to think, been transformed into an educational benediction. I had not foreseen, with my limited perspective, how my action would take on a new meaning within the community.

# Conclusions

In this chapter, there has been a recurring theme of how the larger frame of reference gives a new and deeper meaning to the story of the self that we are inclined to author for ourselves. Our personal narrative is often one that limits who we really are and what we are able to do, for ourselves and others. The woman who was interviewed by Dr Frankl came to see her life as having a new meaning and purpose. The patient who offered a sacramental Polo mint contributed to a narrative of healing in which everyone shared. The laughter over the joke about diarrhoea running in one's jeans united congregation and clergy in a moment of communal hilarity that dispelled the fragmenting and isolating effect of mental illness. And the Good Samaritan story illustrates how often, in unrecognized ways, acts of kindness towards others restore selfhood – and perhaps the realization that the kingdom of Heaven is not situated in some far-off place but right here.

Our unique individual lives are not lessened but enhanced when we see that we all share in the travails of humankind – a greater God-given narrative that invites us to cherish both our uniqueness and our common humanity. Suffering afflicts us all and what cannot be changed must be endured. What is being suggested is that when we really 'hear' another's story and are willing to enter into it, there is the opportunity for a deep paradigm shift to take place. With the help of symbol and metaphor – and sometimes humour — suffering and loss can be framed within a greater, eternal pattern often obscured by mundane concerns. Through this paradigm shift a transcending, universal perspective can be discerned, embracing not only suffering but all of life.

I am also suggesting that a time of crisis can be an opportunity to re-evaluate and change our perspective on life. This is depicted in the Chinese ideogram for crisis, which combines the two characters, danger and opportunity. Perhaps especially in times of danger there is the opportunity to view life through a more universal and eternal perspective, one that brings us closer to God's story as revealed in the seemingly ordinary events of everyday life.

# References

Buber, M. (1958) *I and Thou*. Schribner's.
Carroll, P.L. (1994) *Where God May be Found*. Paulist Press.
Frankl, V. (1984) *Man's Search for Meaning: An Introduction to Logotherapy*. Touchstone, Simon & Schuster.
Reason, P. (2013) *The Sage Handbook of Action Research Participative Inquiry and Practice*. Sage Publications.
Soskice, J.M. (1985) *Metaphor and Religious Language*. Clarendon.
Wilson, M. (1988) *Coat of Many Colours*. Epworth Press.
Yalom, I. (1975) *The Theory and Practice of Group Psychotherapy*. Basic Books.

CHAPTER 12

# Meaning without 'believing': attachment theory, mentalisation and the spiritual dimension of analytical psychotherapy

Jeremy Holmes

This chapter reaches for a psychotherapeutically relevant concept of 'spirituality', outside any specific religious framework. As an 'agnostic atheist', the author identifies with E.M. Forster's 'Oh Lord I disbelieve – help thou my unbelief' (1951), and from that starting point will argue first, that there is a 'spiritual' dimension to psychological health – an aspect of mentalised secure attachment – and second, that this manifests itself in the inner narratives that emerge in successful psychotherapy.

## The phenomenology of therapeutic spirituality

I start with some aspects of psychotherapeutic practice that might usefully be thought as having a spiritual dimension. Three overlapping themes stand out.

### Transcendent experiences

Here is a retrospective account from a 70-year-old psychotherapy patient, for whom an inner 'spiritual' narrative has been a continuing source of comfort through the vicissitudes of his life.

> As a lonely, emotion-suppressed American adolescent on holiday in Europe, he was left to fend for himself while his parents caroused with their friends. He entered Chartres Cathedral and found himself sensing something – as he puts it – 'other, awesome – a direct feeling of the presence of God, which has stayed with me and sustained me ever since'.

In attachment terms, this epiphany could be seen as a response of a habitually avoidant child, a product of Pilgrim Puritanism, to the subliminal (c.f. 'sublime') cues of eternity, grace and ordered complexity implicit in Gothic architecture. The cathedral evoked the presence of a safe, containing, caring Other – the secure base he manifestly lacked. This in turn facilitated the emergence of hitherto inaccessible emotion, a novel and enduring sense of hope and aspiration. The spiritual narrative here typically combines an affect of uplift and care (cf. a mother picking up her crying baby) with a 'God cognition'.

This formulation, as we shall see, is close to the lineaments of secure attachment – subliminal messages that instigate 'broaden and build' states of mind (Granqvist, 2006; Mikulincer & Shaver, 2007). In contrast, Sigmund Freud's famous discussion of *The Uncanny* emphasises the infantile and regressive aspects of transcendent experience. For Freud, omens and portents represent repressed wishes untempered by reality, illustrating 'the omnipotence of thoughts', 'instantaneous wish fulfilments' and 'narcissistic overestimation of subjective mental processes' (Freud, 1919, reprinted 2001a: p. 243).

We now know that paranormal, premonitory and uncanny experiences of the sort undergone by our adolescent protagonist are widespread, and certainly not confined to individuals with mental illness or 'primitives', as was formerly thought (Johns & van Os, 2001). Transcendence needs to be respected and taken seriously. But a distinction needs to be made between the *experiential* legitimacy of these phenomena, and the *explanatory* framework that might account for them (James, 1902). Psychotherapeutic fundamentals include the simultaneous validation of the patient's narrative, combined with tentative probes as to their nature and context. Yeats' couplet (1899) is the therapist's watchword:

> 'I have spread my dreams under your feet
> Tread softly because you tread on my dreams.'

## Ego-less states

Intrinsic to transcendence is a notion of the 'beyond', a realm inaccessible to the conscious, willing, choosing self. Mysticism implies direct contact with the divinity, an infinity beyond everyday experience. Eigen (1998) traces a mystical current in psychoanalytic thinking, drawing particularly on Marion Millner (1987), Winnicott (1962) and Bion (1970), each of whom, in different ways, see the psychotherapeutic encounter and the crucible of the consulting room as a sacred place, providing access to authentic and 'ultimate' psychological reality.

The apotheosis of psychoanalytic mysticism is Bion's (1970) 'O', the impenetrable ground of being from which all knowledge ('K'), desire and memory emanate. Bion links 'O' with 'F', the psychoanalyst's faith in the psychoanalytic process, in life itself and in the capacity to survive destructiveness and attacks on linking. In the consulting room, holding on to hope and communicating in the face of despair that 'this too will pass' is an essential psychotherapeutic attribute.

Two more mundane themes emphasise the importance of ego-less states in therapy. The first is the quotidian mystery of dreaming. However skilful analysts are in unravelling dreams' unconscious meanings, there is always at their core, as Freud acknowledged (1900, reprinted 2001b: p. 525), an impenetrable, un-analysable aspect: 'the dream's navel where it reaches down into the unknown'. As dreamers we cannot fail to be surprised by the complexity, fecundity and strangeness of dream-life. 'How on earth did I think all that up?' we ask ourselves. 'Who is the dreamer that dreams?', 'From whence do dream thoughts come?' – the narrative virtuosity of dream-life remains mysterious despite all the advances in the neuroscience of sleep (Hobson, 2007).

If night dreams are 'spiritual narratives' in the sense that they come from a part of the self not encompassed by the conscious ego, so too do the waking dreams or 'reverie' integral to psychoanalytic work. The therapist must be able to 'dream' lucidly, in the sense of letting her (in this context, 'he' and 'she' are used interchangeably and do not necessarily denote gender) own thoughts and feelings flow impersonally through her, observing them and holding them in readiness for consideration, first with herself and then with the patient.

## *Positive emotions: awe, hope, connectedness*

Jung (1968) saw psychoanalysis as a species of 'alchemy' in which the base metal of neurosis is transformed into psychic gold, or, if we prefer Shakespeare: to 'suffer a sea change/into something rich and strange' (*The Tempest*, Act I, Scene ii, line 565). A therapeutic aim is sublimation, converting symptomatic, repressed or unmodulated sexual and aggressive affect into positive, socially useful or aesthetically pleasing creative enterprises. A patient, troubled by outbursts of unbridled aggression, who can begin to express his feelings through paint or song or dance, is becoming more 'spiritual': less 'driven'; less negative; uplifted rather than brought low; and, as I shall argue, more interpersonally connected.

From this perspective, 'spiritual narratives' have two key features: pro-sociality and relationality. In the heat of the therapeutic relationship, the holding and thoughtfulness of the caregiver distils unbridled and potentially illness-generating affect into constructiveness and connection.

A strong proponent of this perspective is George Vaillant (2008). His argument is threefold:

1   positive emotions are conspicuous by their absence in the psychoanalytic literature
2   narratives of positive emotion have in common an other-directed 'not-me' and/or 'I-Thou' quality, in contrast to the self-preoccupation intrinsic to negative emotions
3   a distinguishing feature of most major religions is the fostering of love, awe, forgiveness, compassion and gratitude.

Vaillant's critique of classical psychoanalysis has to some extent been overtaken by the advent of the 'relational turn' (e.g. Mitchell, 1993), and an increasing number of psychoanalytic publications emphasise the therapeutic role of positive affect (e.g. Akhtar, 2009; Music, 2014). Vaillant's neuroscience perspective suggests that 'spirituality' can be seen as a cluster of positive and pro-social affective and relational phenomena built into our nervous system via the limbic system and the left prefrontal cortex. For him the prosocial emotions of altruism and caregiving have evolutionary survival value and are intrinsically spiritual. However much the content of therapy is concerned with negative emotions – trauma, loss, hate, envy, destructiveness – the therapist's narrative is always one of a positive reaching out to the suffering stranger.

In attempting to explore these issues in more depth, I turn now to findings from attachment theory and especially the work of a group of researchers (Granqvist & Kirkpatrick, 2008) who have attempted to 'ground' spirituality and religion within psychological empiricism.

## Attachment theory and spirituality

The roots of attachment theory lie in Darwinian evolutionary biology (Bowlby, 1990). From this perspective, two general propositions underpin the evolutionary significance of the ubiquity of religion in human societies. First, social groups in which altruism predominates over selfishness tend to have advantages compared with groups in which 'freeloading' and egotism prevail (Boehm, 2012). In most ecologies, social cohesion and collaboration enable groups to overcome more successfully the challenges of existence, such as foraging, reproduction, child-rearing and survival. However, as Freud well knew, humans are also egotistical, narcissistic and nepotistic; these too are necessary for survival in a competitive world, whether that is warring bands of proto-humans or contemporary capitalism (Haidt, 2012). Given that altruism and unselfishness are comparatively weak forces, religious narratives provide vital external reinforcement of positive emotions, a necessary counterbalance to selfishness and devil-take-the-hindmost cultures, and a means of binding groups together (Latin *re-ligare* means 'to bind').

A second point flows from the very fragility of life itself. Attachment theory posits the caregiver/care-seeker relationship as the fundamental basis for security, the psychological analogue of the immune system (Holmes, 2010). What is wrong with death is not death itself since, by secular definition at least, it equates to the cessation of experience. But given the unpredictability both of environments and of social relationships, the capacity of caregivers to protect their loved ones from death and destruction is at best limited; at worst, as in 'disorganised attachment', they are the very source of that deathfulness (Barratt, 2012). There is a permanent vacancy for a deity who can serve as the universal protector, secure base or safe haven – a bulwark against the inescapable facts of death and human destructiveness.

Researchers (Granqvist 2006; Granqvist & Kirkpatrick, 2008; Granqvist *et al*, 2010; Sahdra & Shaver, 2013), using 'attachment narratives' as a framework for researching religion, start from the observation that God has many or all of the features typical of a secure base. These include a relationship with a 'stronger and wiser' being; non-sexual unconditional love; proximity (God is ever-present); a being to whom one can turn at times of extreme danger (as the adage goes, there are 'no atheists in foxholes'); and a reinforcer of positive experiences (blessing marriage, birth, anniversaries, etc.); needed because integral to happiness is its eventual waning or demise and whose disappearance at times of threat and distress evokes extreme mental pain ('My God, my God, why has thou forsaken me?' Psalm 22: 1; Matthew 27: 46).

God's role is to help ease the passage through bereavement, grief and the accompanying emotions of anxiety, depression and despair with far more assurance than is possible for imperfect human caregivers. For social animals the problem of death is loss, experienced and anticipated – loss of one's loved ones, and indeed of one's own existence. To be alone and abandoned is, at least from an infant's perspective, equivalent to death. God can be usefully viewed as an attachment figure, with a vital role to play in the dialectic of loving and losing, which comprises the figured bass of all human life.

## Mystery and mentalising

This approach, based on attachment theory, represents an example of the 'religion is good for you' narrative. Its weakness rests on the assumption that the benefits of belief flow from a deity, rather than the psychological constellation of which the conception of 'God' – leaving entirely aside the question of whether God 'exists' – is a reified symbol. Support for this view comes from Nazi concentration camp survivors. Frankl (2004) noted that 'believers', mainly Orthodox Jews, tended to survive longer in the death camps than those whose beliefs were weak or non-existent. However, the same was also true of atheistic communist inmates whose belief in socialism and the triumph of the proletariat was no less strong. This suggests that it is not what one believes in, but belief itself – an overarching narrative as a source of hope and meaning – that is salutary.

The argument here is that 'spiritual narratives' are good because they 'work' – they keep you sane and healthy, or at least more so than their absence. This position has been criticised by the Anglican Archbishop Rowan Williams (2012). He argues that such 'functionalist' narratives, circumventing the essential ineffability of spirituality, are unwittingly 'secular', further protesting that:

> 'Secularism [...] a functional, instrumentalist perspective, suspicious and uncomfortable about *inaccessible dimensions* – is the hidden mainspring of certain kinds of modern religiousness' (p. 15; italics – J.H.).

I want to link Williams' inaccessible dimensions (the mystery that for him lies at the heart of religion) with the attachment-derived concept of mentalising, or mind-mindedness (Meins, 1997). Before proceeding, I will briefly outline this concept (Allen & Fonagy, 2006; Allen *et al*, 2008; Holmes, 2010).

Mentalising refers to the capacity to stand back from oneself and one's thoughts and to question them. It subsumes notions such as empathy, insight, theory of mind and psychological mindedness, and can be defined as the capacity 'to see oneself from the outside, and others from the inside' (Holmes, 2010). The mentalising perspective includes the following: acceptance that one's perception of the world is inevitably filtered through the mind; that it is therefore subject to error; that one can never fully know another person's mind; and that there are always different versions of reality, or narratives, depending on context. It also argues that relating, through dialogue and exploration, verbal and non-verbal, can lead to a 'fusion of horizons' (Stern, 2010) in which people come to feel empathically linked, one with another and with themselves.

Mentalising is a developmental achievement, not present in infants and small children but gathering pace gradually in course of childhood and adolescence. It is incompatible, however, with extreme anxiety and various states of psychological disturbance. Fonagy and colleagues (2002) identify three 'non-mentalising modes' that developmentally precede mentalising, and that may persist into adult life, especially under adverse developmental conditions.

1. *Teleological thinking* entails an 'if this, then that' viewpoint which bypasses the mind – a psychology based simply on actions and behaviours. Thus, a teleological theology might entail the 'thought' (parenthesised because strictly speaking thoughts do not exist in this mode): 'If I go to Church, I will be safe because God will look after me'.

2. In *equivalence mode* a person makes no distinction between thought and reality, one just 'knows' something to be the case, irrespective of evidence or the 'triangulation' (see Holmes, 2010) that comes from secure interpersonal connectedness. Freud's 'omnipotence of thoughts' (1919, reprinted: 2001a) would be an example of equivalence mode. The fundamentalist conception of scripture as a divine narrative exemplifies equivalence mode.

3. In *pretend mode* the person retreats into, or fails to emerge from, an inner world of fantasy in which the dialectic between thinking and reality is abolished and the external world is viewed as illusory. Many religious phenomena – miracles and mystical experiences – could be seen in terms of pretend mode. Nevertheless, differentiating 'primitive' non-mentalising states from sophisticated mentalising is not always easy. The Buddhist notion of impermanence, which holds that the 'true' nature of reality is an endless cycle of formation and dissolution, might seem (in the face of the apparent solidity of things and people) to be an example of pretend mode. But given what we now know of geological and evolutionary time, of subatomic physics, and neuroscience's failure to find a stable locus for the self among

ever-changing brain states, the impermanence world view may well be more in line with objective reality than our everyday narratives of solidity and stability.

In the light of this, let us return to Williams (2012):

'The non-secular is, foundationally, a willingness to see things or other persons as *the objects of another sensibility than my own*... The point is that what I am aware of, I am aware of as in significant dimensions not defined by my awareness' (p. 13; italics – J.H.)

For Williams, spirituality entails recognizing a viewpoint outside the self, whether this is defined as 'God' or (from my point of view) the unconscious, or the objectivity to which science strives but which because of the limitations of the human mind it can never fully achieve. Williams here is defining 'non-secularity' as a decentring, an acceptance that there are 'more things in heaven and earth' than one's egocentrism would allow. This is in accord with what John Keats wrote (reprinted 2008: p. 277):

'Negative capability, that is when man is capable of being in uncertainties, Mysteries, doubts without any irritable reaching after fact and reason'.

Williams' view is entirely consistent with a scientific world view, in which doubt holds a central place. Writing of art, he says: 'Imaginative construction begins in the sensing of the world in this way, a field of *possible readings*, never therefore reducible to an instrumental account' (Williams, 2012: p. 14; italics – J.H.). This fits well with the notion of mentalising as a species of humility and awe in which one is constantly aware of the limitations and constraints of the mind, and how one's preconceptions and unconscious desires distort experience and relationships.

Equally, the capacity to mentalise is associated with the kinds of favourable developmental experiences that lead one to trust that terrors will be soothed, errors corrected, distress alleviated, and hope that solutions to problems will be found (Allen & Fonagy, 2006). Given this, it comes as no surprise that people with secure attachment have a steadier, more benign and accessible relationship to God, compared with the sudden lurches in and out of faith typical of those with insecure attachment (Granqvist *et al*, 2010).

## Spirituality and psychotherapy

In the light of this possible rapprochement between the attachment-informed psychotherapeutic notion of mentalising and a contemporary religious reading of the non-secular, I want to look at four possible patterns of spirituality in relation to psychotherapy.

### *Spirituality as an alternative to psychotherapy*

The subject of psychotherapy is the realm of the mental. Good therapy outcomes include: enhanced mentalising (Levy *et al*, 2006); the capacity to be more aware of one's emotional and perceptual responses to situations and relationships; the capacity to be more interpersonally sensitive; and the capacity to realise how one's mind makes one the author of one's own destiny, for good or ill. Psychotherapy helps people move from the pre-mentalising narratives described in the preceding section to a more mentalising stance.

However, mentalising can in some circumstances be more bane than boon when action and self-protection, not reflection, are called for. Powerful emotions drive out mentalising (Allen & Fonagy, 2006), whether these be negative (fear, anger and despair) or positive (states of arousal and intense love, sexual or parental). Teleological thinking ('I believe, so all will be well'), equivalence mode ('I *know* that God is on my side') and pretend mode ('My guardian angel will protect me') can all work to keep hope alive and negativity at bay. It would be unhelpful for these beliefs to be mentalised away as being 'just stories/narratives', subject to error and products of adverse developmental experience. Love of God may need to be unquestioning and absolute if it is to work its magic.

In the absence of 'theory of mind', some species of spirituality provide their own route to comfort and survival. Therapists have to steer a delicate course here. Psychotherapy typically aims to help people experience warded-off sadness, depression, anger and anxiety. As Jung (2001: p. 2) put it, before you can lose your self, you have to first find yourself. But challenging absolute beliefs can undermine a person's capacity to maintain hope and be sustained by membership of a supportive community, even though from the perspective of mentalising, not to do so may reinforce denial, encouraging the evacuation of, rather than processing, mental pain.

Mindfulness as an adjunct to psychotherapy (Safran, 2003) illustrates this therapeutic tightrope. Mindfulness-based cognitive therapy (MBCT) is an evidence-based treatment for a number of disorders (Kuyken *et al*, 2010), including recurrent depression. The meditator is encouraged to observe thoughts that arise within, often negative and depressive ones, as 'just thoughts'. To the extent that the content and meaning of the depressive thoughts is discounted, this could be seen as anti-mentalising. On the other hand, to view horrible or traumatic thoughts as 'just thoughts' can also emphasise the role of mind and encourage a decentred, negativity-defusing perspective.

## *Psychotherapy as spirituality*

An important aspect of spirituality is that it often entails regular and sometimes group-based practice – prayer, confession, meditation, church attendance, chanting/singing, imbibing of or smoking sacred substances, or ritualized movement and dance. Typically, these activities take place under the aegis of an older/wiser, revered, endorsed initiate or leader – in the language of attachment theory, someone with secure base features.

Clearly, there is a sense in which regularly attending psychotherapy sessions with a therapist could be seen as a secular analogue of spiritual practice. Indeed, some explicitly make this comparison. In his interview with the author and neurologist Oliver Sacks, Higginbotham (2012) writes:

> 'The relationship with his psychoanalyst, Leonard Shengold, a Manhattan-based Freudian specialist in child abuse and childhood trauma, is one of the most enduring in Sacks's life. In the dedication of *The Man Who Mistook His Wife for a Hat*, Sacks describes Shengold as his mentor; he has seen him twice a week almost every week for 45 years, and continues to do so. "I saw him yesterday," Sacks confirms, "and I'll see him tomorrow".'

Comparably, Alvi, in Woody Allen's film *Annie Hall* quips: 'I'm going to give my psychoanalyst one more year and then I'm going to Lourdes'. As a pragmatic psychiatrist, I see the role of psychotherapy as mutative rather than supportive and I find myself somewhat disapproving of the idea of indefinite therapy. To do so is to blur the boundary between 'God' and 'Caesar'. Jesus, when asked if Jews should pay their taxes to Rome, famously made use of a coin (Matthew 22). In my understanding, psychotherapy belongs firmly to the world of Caesar. Yet in reality the God/Caesar boundary is inherently blurred. I work in a rural area where, despite an increasingly secularized and tolerant-seeming culture, the strict moral values of Methodism are still prevalent. As one patient who had struggled all his life with homosexual feelings put it:

> I've done things my grandparents would have so strongly disapproved of they'd probably have disowned me – where else other than in your consulting room could I talk about these things freely and without censure?

Consistent with the mentalising perspective, the psychotherapeutic narrative in this case could be seen as spiritual (rather than religious) in the sense of its being accepting, non-judgemental and creatively uncertain, offering an otherwise inaccessible degree of comfort and consolation, and validation of autonomy (Holmes & Lindley, 1997).

## *Enhanced spirituality as a psychotherapy outcome*

Psychotherapy defines itself as 'mutative', aiming to produce change. Religious conversion, particularly in its more dramatic or Damascene manifestations, also implies a before-and-after state in which spirituality intervenes in people's lives, rescuing them from despair and setting them on a right(eous) road. Both assume that mutative moments will permeate the personality, affecting not just what happens in the consulting room or place of worship, but more generally transforming a person's attitudes, relationships and way of life.

This 'generalisation' can be seen as enhanced connectedness to hitherto denied or neglected aspects of the self; to other people, especially in one's intimate relationships; but also to society, nature, and ultimately to the universe. Despite disappointment, rage, revenge and the need to retaliate, continuity outweighs loss; one might say that good triumphs over evil. 'Connectedness' and continuity can be seen as spiritual narratives providing a bridge, however fragile, over loss and neglect.

> One patient, nearing the end of 12 years of weekly therapy in which she had sought to overcome a number of 'borderline' features – substance misuse, self-harm, isolation, outbursts of uncontrollable rage, episodes of overwhelming anxiety – reviewed what had, and had not, changed in her life. She still felt unstable and lonely at times, resorting to self-soothing via substance misuse, but she now had a part-time boyfriend and a job, a dog, an allotment, a new house and felt much more connected to her neighbours and small group of friends. She was furious with her therapist for ending, and wanted to walk out without so much as a by-your-leave, but was, with his help, able to tolerate the sadness, turning her feeling of abandonment into a narrative with which she could live. Rather than obliterate him (out-of sight-out-of-mind, as she had felt had been the case with her grossly inadequate parents' behaviour towards her) she was able to feel that her therapist would stay alive within her and that the spirit of what she had gained could endure. Despite her disappointment and loneliness, she felt she was now unlikely to destroy the good things she had achieved in therapy.

## *Spirituality beyond psychotherapy*

Psychotherapy can only take one so far. There comes a point of both liberation and trepidation, where one has to leave the security of one's therapist, her consulting room, and all they represent, and venture into the wider world.

Implicit in enhanced spirituality is a movement from isolation to relatedness, from non-mentalising egocentricity to empathy with the other and oneself. The latter entails the golden rule of reciprocity: 'Do to others as one would have them do to oneself'. From a spiritual perspective the golden rule is not just a covert form of self-interest – the selfish gene knowing which side its bread is buttered. At a fundamental level the other is oneself, made from the same stuff, with the same desires, hopes, fears, vulnerabilities and ambitions, both being in continuity with nature that stretches beyond the merely human.

An important link between Christian spirituality and psychotherapy is contained in the attitude of both to suffering. In his critique of bland post-Christian platitudes offered by neo-religious apologists such as de Botton (2012) and Spufford (2013), Eagleton (2014) reminds us that Christian faith 'is not about moral uplift, political unity or aesthetic charm… It starts from a crucified body' (p. 206).

Vaillant (2008) may bemoan the fact that the psychoanalytic literature focuses more on negative than positive emotions, but surely this is entirely appropriate: alleviating mental pain is the primary rationale for psychoanalytic therapy. The context is always one of hope and trust, but the work entails the identification, experiencing, naming and co-regulation of negative affect.

A typical psychotherapy session might start with the patient feeling 'bad' in some way; the therapist then enters into the maelstrom of this misery and may herself become temporarily infected and affected by it, feeling at times useless and incompetent. But by staying with those feelings, seeing them as grist to the therapeutic mill, as representing an aspect of the patient's inner world – feelings too painful perhaps for the patient to have faced on their own – patient and therapist then work together to encompass these 'bad' feelings in a framework of mutual understanding. Finally, there will be a lightening, a sense of a movement from dark into the light, glimmers of hope and even pleasure; a job done, hand-to-hand, collaboratively.

Psychotherapy assumes that facing mental pain, rather than sequestering it or overlaying it with false hope and reassurance, is the true route to transformation. A similar ethic is central to the Christian notion of sacrifice: Christ suffers with and for humankind, and thereby our burden is lightened. This can be compared with the co-regulation of affect that is a central part of the parental role and which, when performed sensitively and responsively, forms the foundation for secure attachment (Slade & Holmes, 2014). One of the ultimate forms of suffering people can experience is a parent's loss of their child; by 'sacrificing' his own son (as he had earlier asked Abraham to do), God enters this human world of near-unendurable pain.

In Buddhism suffering is also centre-stage. Prince Gautama's confrontation with poverty, disease and death led him to abandon his golden-boy protected life and seek enlightenment and simplicity. Buddhism's central paradox is that the first step towards release from suffering is acceptance that suffering is inevitable. This too is consistent with the psychotherapeutic ethos. Suffering here links with the notion of 'impermanence': everything – living and non-living – is subject to change; our conception of fixed entities, including mental pain itself, is illusory. This idea is vital for therapists, especially when working with minds *in extremis*. The hope implicit in the therapeutic narrative of Buddhism is that however awful one feels at any given moment, impermanence means that today's misery will look different in tomorrow's light.

## Non-attachment

Staying with Buddhist narratives, Shadra & Shaver (2013) and others (e.g. Holmes, 1997; Safran, 2003) have noted the conceptual proximity (despite the linguistic discrepancy) of the Buddhist notion of non-attachment and secure attachment. In Buddhist theology non-attachment might appear to imply affective withdrawal, seeming self-sufficiency or splendid isolation, states that in attachment terms would be classified as detachment, avoidance or deactivation.

However, non-attachment can be viewed as the ability to occupy the middle ground, to take into account all possible perspectives, including the certainty that one will at times be wrong, to give one's hopes and desires and longings their due but without succumbing to blind pursuit of ever-elusive certainties. Non-attachment is an affirmation of the ever-changing nature of existence, a liberation from stasis and rigidity.

Attachment theory similarly emphasises the fluid and seamless capacity of securely attached children to handle both attachment and separation. Secure adults can accept loss as the obverse of connection and adapt to the circumstances in which they find themselves without conformism or compliance. A degree of healthy detachment may be needed when faced with rebuff, and a measure of clinging when inconsistency threatens, but a secure individual retains the ability to stay grounded, having an ultimate confidence in relationship and being aware of the dangers of isolation. The idea of disorganized attachment represents the ultimate in relational disruption and destructiveness. People with secure attachment, as well as those with non-attachment, know that 'disorganization' is never far away; we live on the edge of chaos, socially, individually, biologically, and yet refuse to despair or give up. Nor do we perversely celebrate and augment chaos.

Freud (1933, reprinted: 2001c) proudly claimed that his discovery of the power of the unconscious and the converse limitations of the conscious mind, was, after Galileo and Darwin, the third of the great science-led blows to man's narcissism. People seek therapy because they want to 'change', but paradoxically change comes about only to the extent that we can accept ourselves, and feel accepted as we are (see Linehan *et al*, 2006). Our capacity to modify our destiny depends on being able to accept our weakness, vulnerability, helplessness, in Freud's terms our 'castratedness' (Barratt, 2012). Contra Rousseau, we are not born free, but find ourselves held everywhere within the chains of our family and social history.

By transforming pain into narrative, whether spiritual or psychotherapeutic, a degree of emotional freedom is possible. Freedom flows, paradoxically, from the creative use of constraint. As Dylan Thomas (1957) so beautifully puts it in *Fern Hill*:

> 'Time held me green and dying
> Though I sang in my chains like the sea.'

The role of psychotherapy is to foster the capacity to understand and give narrative voice to the constraints of which we are a product, and find ways to forgive ourselves and others; to live in a present moment imbued with 'spirit', which is always relational with the other, with the natural world, and with ourselves. Psychotherapy helps us sing in our chains.

## Conclusions

Implicit in attachment research (Mikulincer & Shaver, 2007) is a valuation of the role of the 'higher' spiritual values of love, connectedness and care.

People with secure attachment, and those with insecure attachment who are exposed to positive narratives, are more likely to manifest 'goodness' – altruism, anti-xenophobia, creativity and compromise – than people with insecure attachment. This inherently 'top-down', non-reductionist viewpoint is implicit in the spiritual narratives that psychotherapy can foster (Ellis, 2008). At first glance this position appears incompatible with a psychoanalytic approach based on psychic determinism, in which psychic life is primarily under the sway of the unconscious. Notably, the attachment model of love, characterised by mentalising, acknowledgement and protective feelings for the other contrasts with Freud's equation of love with erotic drive discharge and liberation from the oppressive influence of the anti-libidinal superego.

Contemporary psychoanalytic approaches suggest that Freud's model is outdated. The unconscious is a source of creative possibility, embodying our evolutionary heritage. Spiritual values help eliminate, select and channel the best of all that is thrown up from 'below'. As a therapist, one listens to one's unconscious – including the base desires with which one might wish to exploit, seduce or punish one's patients – and then with the help of spirituality first acknowledges and then recruits these feelings in the service of love (Holmes, 2014a). Acceptance of negative affect, without being blinded by it, is intrinsic to truth-seeking (Cassidy, 1994). Spirituality reflects the 'benign superego' (Holmes, 2014b), without which we and our patients would be condemned to inhabit a Hobbesian world of nastiness, brutishness and brevity.

Coming from a position of agnostic atheism, this chapter has been informed by three basic principles. First, spiritual narratives cannot be thought of as a separate realm beyond the bio-psychosocial perimeter of psychotherapeutic practice. For a psychotherapist, no aspect of human life, however 'negative', is alien: either everything or nothing is sacred. Second, no consulting room is an island, for human psychology is part of a web of connections and patterns that extend through intimate relationships to the non-human living world and into the inanimate sphere of the material universe. Third, humans are blessed (and perhaps cursed) with the ability not only to suffer joy and misery but also to reflect on those experiences. This mentalising vantage point is itself a product of evolution-driven developmental processes. When things go well, caregivers' reflexivity enables them to pass on that capacity to their offspring; much of the work of psychotherapy is concerned with trying to re-establish this developmental track in people for whom it has gone awry.

Mentalising can be thought of as spiritual in two ways, philosophical and ethical. Because Rowan Williams' 'inaccessibility' is intrinsic to the idea of mentalising, the error-prone, self-constrained mind can never fully apprehend the mystery of the thing-in-itself; one of psychotherapy's prime tasks is to help people accept uncertainty and the irony of the freedom it bestows. Mentalising is also spiritual in the ethical sense that it implies a degree of non-attachment: the capacity to lean away from oneself (Holmes, 2014a), to view suffering – one's own and others' – with equanimity and compassion, and to activate the 'top-down' values needed for its alleviation. From the attachment perspective, psychotherapy is no more and no less than an intensely practical and loving pathway to spiritual aliveness.

# References

Akhtar, S. (ed.) (2009) *Good Feelings: Psychoanalytic Reflections on Positive Attitudes and Emotions*. Karnac.
Allen, J. & Fonagy, P. (eds) (2006) *Handbook of Mentalisation-Based Treatment*. Wiley.
Allen, J., Fonagy, P. & Bateman, A. (2008) *Mentalising in Clinical Practice*. American Psychiatric Publishing.
Barratt, B. (2012) *What is Psychoanalysis?* Routledge.
Bion, W. (1970) *Attention and Interpretation*. Tavistock.
Boehm, C. (2012) *Moral Origins: The Evolution of Virtue, Altruism and Shame*. Basic Books.
Bowlby, J. (1990) *Charles Darwin: A New Biography*. Hutchinson.
Cassidy, J. (1994) Emotion regulation: influence of attachment relationships. *Monographs of the Society for Research in Child Development*, **59**, 228–83.
de Botton, A. (2012) *Religion for Atheists: A Non-Believer's Guide to the Uses of Religion*. Hamish Hamilton.
Eagleton, T. (2014) *Culture and the Death of God*. Yale University Press.
Eigen, M. (1998) *The Psychoanalytic Mystic*. Free Association Books.
Ellis, G. (2008) *Faith, Hope & Doubt in Times of Uncertainty*. Quakers Australia.
Fonagy, P., Gergely, G., Jurist, E., et al (2002) *Affect Regulation, Mentalisation, and the Development of the Self*. Other Press.
Forster, E.M. (1951) What I believe. In *Two Cheers for Democracy* (ed. E.M. Forster). Arnold.
Frankl, V. (2004) *Man's Search For Meaning*. Random House.
Freud, S. (2001a) The Uncanny (1919). In *The Standard Edition of the Complete Psychological Works of Sigmund Freud*. Vol. 17: An Infantile Neurosis and Other Works (ed. & transl. J. Strachey). Vintage Classics.
Freud, S. (2001b) The interpretation of dreams (1900). In *The Standard Edition of the Complete Psychological Works of Sigmund Freud*. Vol. 5 (ed. & transl. J. Strachey). Vintage Classics.
Freud, S. (2001c) *The Standard Edition of the Complete Psychological Works of Sigmund Freud*. Vol. 22: New Introductory Lectures on Psycho-Analysis and Other Works (ed. & transl. J. Strachey). Vintage Classics.
Granqvist, P. (2006) On the relation between secular and divine relationships: an emerging attachment perspective and a critique of the 'depth' approaches. *International Journal for the Psychology of Religion*, **16**, 1–18.
Granqvist, P. & Kirkpatrick, L. (2008) Attachment and religious representations and behaviour. In *Handbook of Attachment* (eds J. Cassidy & P. Shaver). Guilford Press.
Granqvist, P., Mikulincer, M. & Shaver, P. (2010) Religion as attachment: normative processes and individual differences. *Personality and Social Psychology Review*, **14**, 49–61.
Haidt, J. (2012) *The Righteous Mind: Why Good People are Divided by Politics and Religion*. Allen Lane.
Higginbotham, A. (2012) Oliver Sacks' most mind-bending experiment. *The Telegraph*, 12 October. Available at http://www.telegraph.co.uk/books/authors/oliver-sacks-most-mind-bending-experiment/ (accessed 9 November 2015).
Hobson, A. (2007) Wake up or dream on? Six questions for Turnbull and Solms. *Cortex*, **43**, 1113–15.

Holmes, J. (1997) *Attachment, Intimacy, Autonomy*. Jason Aronson.
Holmes, J. (2010) *Exploring in Security: Towards an Attachment-informed Psychoanalytic Psychotherapy*. Routledge.
Holmes, J. (2014a) *The Therapeutic Imagination: How Literature can Deepen Psychodynamic Understanding and Enhance Empathy*. Routledge.
Holmes, J. (2014b) *Attachments: Psychotherapy, Psychiatry, Psychoanalysis*. Routledge.
Holmes, J. & Lindley, R. (1997) *The Values of Psychotherapy*, 2nd edn. Karnac Books.
James, W. (1902) *The Varieties of Religious Experience: A Study in Human Nature*. Reprinted: 2008. Folio Society.
Johns, L. & van Os, J. (2001) The continuity of psychotic experience in the general population. *Clinical Psychology Review*, **21**, 1125–46.
Jung, C.G. (1968) *Psychology and Alchemy*. Volume 12 of the Collected Works of C.G. Jung. Princeton University Press.
Jung, C.G. (2001) *Modern Man in Search of a Soul*. Routledge.
Keats, J. (2008) *The Complete Poetical Works and Letters of John Keats, Cambridge Edition*. Read Country Books.
Kuyken, W., Watkins, E., Holden, E., et al (2010) How does mindfulness based therapy work? *Behaviour Research and Therapy*, **48**, 1105–12.
Levy, K., Clakin, J., Yeomans, F., et al (2006) Mechanisms of change in the treatment of borderline personality disorder treated with transference focused psychotherapy. *Journal of Clinical Psychology*, **62**, 481–501.
Linehan, M., Comtois, K., Murray, A., et al (2006) Two-year randomised controlled trial and follow-up of Dialectical Behaviour Therapy vs therapy by experts for suicidal behaviours and borderline personality disorder. *Archives of General Psychiatry*, **63**, 757–66.
Meins, E. (1997) *Security of Attachment and the Development of Social Cognition*. Psychology Press.
Mikulincer, M. & Shaver, P. (2007) *Attachment in Adults*. Guilford Press.
Millner, M. (1987) *The Suppressed Madness of Sane Men*. Tavistock.
Mitchell, S. (1993) *Hope and Dread in Psychoanalysis*. Basic Books.
Music, G. (2014) *The Good Life: Wellbeing and the New Science of Altruism, Selfishness, and Immorality*. Routledge.
Safran, J. (ed.) (2003) *Psychoanalysis and Buddhism: An Unfolding Dialogue*. Wisdom.
Sahdra, B. & Shaver, P. (2013) Comparing attachment theory and Buddhist psychology. *International Journal for the Psychology of Religion*, **23**, 282–93.
Shakespeare, W. (1968) *The Tempest*. Nonesuch Press.
Slade, A. & Holmes, J. (eds) (2014) Introduction. In *Attachment Theory*. Sage.
Spufford, F. (2013) *Unapologetic: Why, Despite Everything, Christianity Can Still Make Surprising Emotional Sense*. Bloomsbury.
Stern, D. (2010) *Partners in Thought: Working with Unformulated Experience, Dissociation, and Enactment*. Routledge.
Thomas, D. (1957) 'The force that through the green fuse drives the flower'. In *Collected Poems*. Faber.
Vaillant, G. (2008) *Spiritual Evolution: How We are Wired for Faith, Hope and Love*. Broadway Books.
Williams, R. (2012) *Faith in the Public Square*. Bloomsbury.
Winnicott, D. (1962) *The Maturational Processes and the Facilitating Environment*. Hogarth.
Yeats, W.B. (1899) 'Aedh Wishes for the Cloths of Heaven'. In *Wordsworth Poetry Library: Collected Poems of WB Yeats*. Reprinted: 2008. Wordsworth.

CHAPTER 13

# Stories of living with loss: spirituality and ageing

John Wattis and Steven Curran

Loss occurs throughout life but is often concentrated in old age. However, late life can also be seen as a time of positive personal development when new conflicts are resolved. Development is a dynamic process which may occur whenever an individual faces challenges, including the challenges of loss. Many old people cope with these losses with amazing resilience. Where do narrative and spirituality come into this? Indeed, what are narrative and spirituality in this context?

## Narrative in context

The idea of narrative in medical practice and research has 'come of age'. Listening to people's stories is an essential part of holistic care. Reflecting on this, we remember how the interpersonal aspects of healthcare have always been as important as the technical aspects. We have advised students when taking a history with a 'difficult' patient to drop the schema of the medical history and try to simply listen empathetically to the patient telling their story. This is a skill that is often acquired only after years of practice. The standard psychiatric history nevertheless forms a focused schema for efficiently ensuring that all relevant parts of the story are heard, and the old-fashioned psychiatric formulation is still important as a way of ensuring that all relevant aspects of the narrative are considered before a care or management plan is developed.

Narrative has also to be set in the context of the world view and mindset of the individual patient and practitioner. World views have to do with the presuppositions that shape the thinking and activity of members of a culture or society. Wright (1992) states: 'Wherever we find the ultimate concerns of human beings we find world views' (p. 122). According to Wright, world views characteristically do four things: they provide stories (or narratives) through which people view reality; these stories help to define and answer the basic questions of human existence; they are associated with a series of cultural symbols; and they provide praxis, a 'way-of-being-in-the-world' that derives from the narrative and how it addresses fundamental questions of the culture. Culture itself is largely expressed through praxis and symbol (often without a conscious reference to the controlling narrative). For a more detailed exposition of world view in a theological context, the reader is referred to Wright (1992: pp. 122–126).

In old-age mental health, it has always been important to understand the problem the patient is presenting in the light of their physical, family and social context, as well as being aware that patients have their own 'take' on what is important and that their story needs interpreting in the light of their own experiences and culture. Not only that, we live in a multicultural society and different cultures may have different 'controlling narratives' reflected in different world views and mindsets. To develop spiritual competence, the healthcare practitioner needs not only to become aware of their own world view and mindset but also to be sensitive to differences between individual patients, generations and cultural groups. This includes differences of world view between members of the therapeutic team, which may lead to inefficiency and potential conflict. For those working in organisations such as the National Health Service there is also the tricky question of the (not always benign) organisational culture to consider.

## What is meant by spirituality?

A standard theological text (McGrath, 2011) candidly states: 'The term is resistant to precise definition... However, it is clear that spirituality is *generally* understood to mean the experiencing of God and the transforming of lives as a result of that experience' (p. 109; italics – authors'). Writing in the context of affective disorders in late life, Dew & Koenig (2008) contrasted religion with spirituality, describing religion as referring to a collection of beliefs and behaviours embraced by a group, and spirituality as a more personal search for a relationship with the transcendent, not necessarily institutionally related. A fuller discussion of the definition of spirituality and the definition used in this book (Cook, 2004) is found in Chapter 1, 'Narrative in psychiatry, theology and spirituality' (p. 5). This embraces the possibility of a 'secular' as well as a God-centred 'sacred' view of spirituality and sits better in a pluralistic culture than some other definitions that see spirituality purely as relating to God.

Whether sacred or secular, spirituality has profound significance for clinical practice. Gordon *et al* (2011) point out that 'The key to providing spiritual care is to understand what spirituality means to the person you are caring for' (p. 5). Kang (2003) usefully describes six dimensions of spirituality that inform spiritually competent healthcare and on which we shall be drawing.

1 Becoming: volitionally directed growth of the self through 'active doing'.
2 Meaning: the sense of intrinsic purposefulness and vitality rooted in personal, collective or transpersonal spaces.

3   Being: a pervasive quality that forms the foundation of our existence as human beings.
4   Centredness: an inner stability based on knowing and recognising what lies at the core of one's being.
5   Connectedness: seeing the self as a 'fluid process' embedded within a larger interrelational context.
6   Transcendence: the innate human drive to find ultimate meaning and happiness and the goal that this drive seeks.

'Active doing' means active engagement in activities that are purposeful.

## Resilience and living with loss

The well-established model of psychosocial development put forward by Erikson (1965) regards the core conflict of the last stage of life as being between 'ego integrity and despair'. Success in this struggle can be seen as giving meaning to loss in late life. The biggest loss to be faced is loss of one's own life. There are many interesting reflections on how the tasks of later life are viewed and faced in different religious traditions (see Jewell, 1999). However, in mental healthcare we must always seek to understand and support each individual's own unique mindset, quest for meaning, purpose and connectedness, and we must be aware how they relate to our own, so as not to impose, consciously or unconsciously, our own values on the patient.

## Transitions and losses associated with ageing

Old age requires the individual to adapt to a number of transitions, not all of which should be classed as losses. There is, for example, the joy of becoming a grandparent or later, a great-grandparent. There are other transitions such as retirement which can be seen in part as loss (e.g. of work colleagues, income and status) and in part as gain (e.g. more time to spend on enjoyable interests that have been suppressed by the demands of working life). Bereavement, though not confined to old age, certainly becomes more common with increasing age, especially in higher-income societies where most people survive into old age. There may be loss of physical fitness, perhaps associated with the development of chronic, limiting physical illness and infirmity. Often there is a loss of income, sometimes loss of independence, autonomy and control, and ultimately, the loss of life in death. Loss of memory and self-control in dementia is something that many older people worry about, though paradoxically personal concern about memory loss is perhaps more common in those with depression than those with dementia. For a wider consideration of spirituality in dementia see Wallace (2011).

This chapter will explore narratives of loss faced by people as they age, how they cope and how they may be assisted by spiritually competent practitioners. We will consider this from the broad perspective of Cook's definition, looking for how the quest for meaning, purpose and connectedness relates to successful coping. The narratives are fictionalised but based on real-life encounters that we and other members of the Spirituality Special Interest Group at the University of Huddersfield have had with older patients.

We will start with a narrative of a 'model case' developed by our colleagues (Jones *et al*, 2016) for their concept analysis of spirituality in occupational therapy.

## Narrative 1. Jean: coping with stroke

>Jean was a 67-year-old woman with short-term memory problems, which she tried to overcome using various strategies. She had had a stroke 6 months after her husband's death, and had then sold her home and moved to a ground floor apartment with a small garden. Her interests included gardening, playing the piano, spending time with her family and participating in the Women's Institute's activities. Piano playing was a strategy she used to reduce her anxiety.
>
>The stroke had left Jean with right-sided weakness of upper and lower limbs. From an acute hospital ward she was transferred to an intermediate care residential setting for 6 weeks' rehabilitation. The focus was to improve her independence with activities of daily living and to reduce her dependence on a care package when she was discharged home. Jean's goals were identified in collaboration with the occupational therapist. She needed to plan a new life for herself in her new home without her husband, and come to terms with the loss of function and cognitive capacities following the stroke. The spiritual theme of 'becoming' that person was a key concept for her to convey to those who provided her therapy and care. Achieving a sense of personal independence and satisfaction with her life was an important aspect of her being. She had meaningful and purposeful hobbies (gardening and playing the piano) but they required some adaptation before she was able to enjoy them. Connecting with her family and community were important aspects of Jean's spiritual well-being. She was motivated to remain an active member of both and also of her faith community.
>
>Jean worked with her occupational therapist to develop an inner resilience to overcome her anxiety and to develop practical strategies to cope. Playing the piano helped her manage her anxiety, and she drew strength from her faith and belief in God.

The many different aspects of Jean's improved well-being included all of Kang's six dimensions. This can be taken as an example of achieving healing and 'wholeness', mediated by a spiritually aware practitioner, in the face of the disintegrating pressures of personal loss and illness.

## Narrative 2. Maureen: coping with depression

>Maureen was admitted to the old-age psychiatry ward with a severe episode of recurrent depression. She was 65 years old and on this occasion had been depressed for 4 years; she had only recently been discharged from another

psychiatric unit. She was almost mute, it was difficult to get her to eat or drink and she was losing weight. Her husband, who had retired 5 years earlier, was worn out with looking after her. The marital relationship had deteriorated into recrimination on the one side and silence on the other.

The couple had a daughter and grandchildren of whom Maureen was very fond and with whom she had been closely involved, but 3 years previously they had been rehoused 5 miles away and as her depression progressed, Maureen stopped trying to get to see them. She did not even respond when they were brought to see her. Maureen had previously been a keen member of the local Anglican Church but her involvement there had stopped as her depression deepened and she had turned away attempts by her co-religionists to reach out to her.

On the ward her refusal to eat, drink or take medication necessitated a course of electroconvulsive therapy (ECT) as a life-saving measure. Although her depression improved, she remained rather apathetic and staff noted a somewhat hostile reaction when her husband visited. The team psychologist met them and explored the marital interaction. The husband was critical of his wife and she for her part was resentful of the way that he had taken over household duties from her (as she saw it, to fill in his spare time since his retirement). Marital therapy was instituted and work was also done on repairing the relationship with her daughter. Eventually, Maureen was discharged home and remained well, but she still missed being close to her grandchildren, who (as she put it) had given a meaning and purpose to her life. With help, she and her husband managed to move nearer the daughter and Maureen resumed her role of a grandmother, helping to look after the kids when her daughter was at work. She also spontaneously resumed church attendance, becoming once more a committed member of her faith community.

Some people would see the 'spiritual' part of this as Maureen resuming attendance at church but in our analysis it is the sense of meaning and purpose in life, the mending of relationships with her family, and the increased sense of connectedness and purpose that are the main indicators of 'spiritually competent' care. This was achieved by taking into account all the relevant factors in Maureen's story: the presence of a genetic tendency to recurrent depression, the loss of role related to her husband's retirement and his 'takeover' at home, and the loss of contact with the grandchildren. Maureen's worsening depression and withdrawal all contributed to the situation and interacted with each other in a negative way such that Maureen very nearly lost her 'being'. Elements of becoming, regaining meaning, being, centredness, connectedness, transcendence (Kang, 2003) and the endurance and ultimate resolution of suffering (Jones *et al*, 2016) can all be seen in this narrative, which concluded with the re-engagement with religious practice and reconnection with Maureen's church community. Merely treating the presenting problem of severe depression with ECT and medication, although necessary, would have been unlikely to lead to a long-term resolution of her illness without the other interventions described. Last, Maureen's re-engagement with her family and her religion may have helped reduce the risk of future relapse.

## Narrative 3. Janet: coping with bereavement and loss of role

Janet, a 73-year-old single lady with a history of anxiety, consulted the advanced nurse practitioner at her doctor's surgery after her 94-year-old mother died. Janet had been the main carer for her mother and had never married, moving in with her mother for the last few years of her life. Her mother had been very domineering and critical of Janet, who rarely went out and took intermittent medication for severe anxiety. Janet was socially very isolated and had noticed that her anxiety had risen.

Janet was angry at her mother for having dominated her life and for dying. She did not belong to any faith community and found no consolation in ideas about God. She felt there was no purpose to her life. The nurse spent a number of consultations with Janet listening to her concerns and fears about her anxiety and her life.

Janet used to enjoy gardening but this had stopped when she moved in with her mother. The nurse introduced Janet to a local mental health charity worker who taught pottery at a community project. Janet joined this group and also found out about a gardening group which met at the same centre twice a week. Over a number of months she started to become more involved in pottery and gardening and started to gain confidence in relating to others and going out of the flat. After 6 months she became a volunteer at the centre serving at their community café.

Janet found a sense of meaning and purpose through the community projects and volunteering work. She told the nurse that working with the mental health charity had given her new insight into how to deal with anxiety and she realised how isolated she had become and how her self-esteem had suffered because of her mother's behaviour.

Again, elements of 'becoming' (the will to choose and enact a new role), meaning, being, centredness, connectedness and overcoming suffering can be seen in this account. Although the element of transcendence is arguably missing, some would recognise it in Janet's finding meaning and happiness through her volunteering.

## Narrative 4. David: loss beyond endurance

David was admitted to an old-age psychiatric in-patient ward following a period of low mood. Five years earlier he had retired from the fire and rescue service after completing the maximum 30 years' service. During his working life he had been a dedicated fireman who worked his way through the ranks to become chief fire officer. He had been decorated for bravery several times and had been regularly asked to give advice on fire and rescue management at local and national governmental levels.

Following retirement, David's sense of meaning and purpose diminished and his motivation to participate in other activities was minimal. His marriage broke down and his wife of 35 years applied for a divorce 6 months before his admission as he 'was not the man he used to be'. As a result, he had to leave his large semi-rural family home to live in a small apartment nearer town. David had also been recently diagnosed with heart failure and an exacerbation of a work-related breathing problem that had resulted in him breathing in noxious fumes, damaging his lungs.

On the ward, David regularly spoke about how he once 'was somebody' and how after retirement the loss of his status 'destroyed my life and meaning as a man'. He missed the comradeship of his workmates and the power he had as a fire officer, making life-and-death decisions in emergency situations. He explained how he missed his family home, which was situated on top of a hill, allowing him to look over the valleys to the other hills, 'grounding' him and making him feel 'free and part of the world'. He talked about the wind on his face and the extreme 'power' of the weather and what it could do. He mentioned little about his estranged wife and daughter.

David's wife reported that in retrospect she felt he was actually 'married to the job' and had been a rather distant figure in both her and their daughter's lives. She had looked forward to his retirement, thinking that it would be 'our time, now', hoping they could have a long and happy life together. However, from the day he retired he had become emotionally distant, intolerant of her at best and at worst physically abusive. She said the violence had never happened before but she could not live with the fear of it happening again in the future.

Despite intensive treatment of his depression and psychological support, David's mood deteriorated and he began to express suicidal intentions. He was focused on his loss of role as chief fire officer and the loss of the value he felt for himself, and he could see no purpose for his future existence. He regularly said he was not needed any more because he could no longer save lives. He stated 'I used to be the hero'. This theme was explored further with David's nurse and he began to agree that there were other ways to save lives or help others that did not have to include the drama of a rescue, which David had emphasised as part of his sense of loss. Further conversations with him concerned his feelings of grounding when he used to be in his garden. A trip was arranged to a local area of beauty among the hills to see if he could sense the same feelings and connection with the world he used to have, and which might enhance his spiritual well-being. Because of the assessed risk, David had to be accompanied on these visits, although he had wanted to be alone, since it was the solitude and communion with the natural world he craved.

As time went on, David's mood began to improve and he gained motivation to return home to begin a new chapter in his life. Eventually, after periods of leave from hospital, he was discharged to the care of a community mental health team (CMHT).

Two weeks later the in-patient team received information from the CMHT that David had tragically died by suicide. In a letter left explaining his reasons, he thanked the mental health team for trying but wrote he could not live any longer and that his 'real' life had ended the day he retired. He did, however, say that although the visits to local areas of beauty did not achieve what the team had hoped for, they allowed him to make his peace with God for the first time and die at the time that was 'right' for him.

All relevant physical treatments had been given, the suicide risk had been assessed and managed carefully, yet the patient still died. What about the management of David's spiritual needs? How far could the six dimensions (becoming, meaning, being, centredness, connectedness, transcendence) and overcoming suffering be addressed? David had suffered multiple losses: of role, of his marriage, of his beloved home, of his physical prowess. His sense of personal worth and meaning had centred on his work and he never really found anything that could take their place. In that sense he had not managed to become the person he needed to be to survive. David had also lost much of his connectedness with work colleagues and family. Yet he had found a partial reconnection with transcendence through his visits to the country.

The note David left saying that he had made peace with God for the first time and that he had died at the time that was 'right' for him suggests that his spiritual needs had been met in part, but could more have been done? Would he have died a more tortured soul had he not had the support? These are the questions that practitioners ask themselves. The nurse who was involved with David says she still asks herself from time to time whether they could have done more, or whether this man's feeling that he had made peace with God was the best they could have jointly achieved.

## *Narrative 5. Margaret and George: coping with dementia*

Margaret, 76 and George, 78, had been married for over 50 years. George, previously a farmer, felt well although he did admit that his memory 'wasn't as good as it used to be'. Margaret agreed that George's memory had been getting gradually worse but she also explained that now he regularly misplaced things such as his glasses, car keys and wallet and accused her of stealing his things, which led arguments and distress for both. George was sleeping poorly and Margaret was not getting enough sleep either. When first referred, Margaret herself felt stressed and low in mood.

George and Margaret were initially assessed at home by the memory service nurse. Margaret's concerns were also discussed. George was reasonably well from a physical perspective and taking no prescribed medications, although his spectacles 'needed checking'. Margaret had been gathering facts about George's illness and had come to the view that 'it looks like dementia'. Further investigations and a medical assessment confirmed Alzheimer's disease. Initially Margaret seemed relieved by the diagnosis and she expressed a determination 'to beat it by every means possible'. Margaret quickly became, in her words, an 'expert' on dementia. She pushed for George to be started on an anti-dementia drug. She arranged for his GP to undertake a physical health review and booked an eye test for new spectacles. Understanding the importance of George's physical health, she arranged for a male helper to take George out every day for a long walk and for some 'male company'. All her thoughts and energy were focused on George. After a few months, things seemed to stabilise and even improve slightly.

Over the next 4 years George deteriorated to the point where he was unable to recall the names of family members and friends and needed help with all his day-to-day needs. Margaret was finding caring for him increasingly stressful. She was not getting enough sleep and described herself as 'shattered'. Eventually she took the painful decision to move George into a care home, although she felt guilty about this.

The same doctor had been involved throughout her journey as a carer and Margaret was able to form a trusting relationship with him. As George's illness progressed, she eventually felt able to discuss her concerns and worries about the future. In 'losing' her husband, a good friend and her physical and emotional security for the future, she was left feeling devastated and frightened.

Once George had moved into a care home, Margaret was able to slowly recover. Looking back and reflecting on her role as a carer, she felt relieved that 'everything that could be done had been done'. She took the decision after very careful consideration and discussion to 'stop dwelling on the past' and 'what I've lost' and to stop 'worrying about the future'. She wanted to 'get the most out of every day'. She felt more emotionally intimate with George and she was able to enjoy a simple smile or word; she particularly cherished just holding hands.

George was very settled in the care home, which was run along the lines of 'person-centred care' advocated by the School of Dementia Studies at the University of Bradford (www.bradford.ac.uk/health/dementia/dementia-care-mapping), and Margaret got a lot of comfort from this. She assisted George with his meals and his day-to-day needs, spending time in the garden with him and befriending other residents and carers. In the latter stages of George's illness the focus was on helping Margaret to make sense of things and what their life together meant. For Margaret, George's illness was initially a devastating loss, but eventually this was seen as bringing them closer together emotionally. Margaret also had a much greater appreciation of 'the important things in life'. Although not a religious person, Margaret felt 'at peace'.

This story shows Margaret going through several stages of 'becoming'. She initially addressed the suffering of seeing her husband develop dementia by becoming 'an expert'. Later, when he had to move into residential care, she became a companion in the 'eternal present moment' of his dementia. She found meaning in the wonderful life they had shared and, she felt, continued to share. She was supported in this by her doctor and the memory team but she also developed connectedness with other residents and carers in the residential home. She overcame the distress of the previous 6 years and became centred in her new role, developing an appreciation of what was important in life for her.

George's story is harder to tell. Although there are accounts of the experience of dementia by people in early stages of illness (see Saunders, 2013), the experiences of people at later stages have to be inferred partly from their behaviour and partly from observational methods such as Dementia Care Mapping (www.bradford.ac.uk/health/dementia/dementia-care-mapping). There is research evidence that Dementia Care Mapping acts as a measure of both quality of care and quality of life and that, used within an organisational framework that supports patient-centred care, it can improve levels of well-being, increase the diversity of occupation and decrease the incidence of personal detractions (Brooker, 2005). In essence, carers need to develop compassionate understanding of the person being cared for. This can be encouraged through exercises such as Dementia Care Mapping but also by the provision of objects of personal significance or life history books around which carers and the person cared for can reminisce. The assembling of such objects or the making of a life history book for guidance can be an activity for people with mild or moderate dementia to share with family and friends and can be a continuing link into the person's history, interests and personal sense of meaning as dementia progresses. Resources for people with dementia and their carers, including advice on developing a life history book, are availabe, for example, at the Alzheimer's Society website (www.alzheimers.org.uk). This can include any religious observance or other activity with spiritual significance for the patient. We well remember a lady with quite advanced dementia who used to be brought to her local Quaker meeting for worship by friends or family and who would sit in contented silence throughout the meeting.

People ask 'What happens to the spirit in advanced dementia?' We can give no definite answer. However, if we look at the related phenomenon of personhood, it seems that as dementia advances, so our personal experience of well-being becomes increasingly dependent on those around us validating us as individuals (Kitwood, 1997). Thus, it is reasonable to assume that the spiritual well-being of people with dementia likewise becomes increasingly dependent on others, placing considerable responsibility on those (often under-trained, over-busy and under-supported) care staff who look after many old people with severe dementia.

## *Narrative 6. Ibrahim: coping with loss and poverty in Pakistan*

Ibrahim was a 65-year-old man assessed by a nurse in outreach practice in Pakistan. He had been out of work for 20 years despite his best efforts, including an unsuccessful attempt to start a small business. By Western standards he was living in poverty. He had had diabetes for some years but kept his blood sugar well controlled by diet. He had also had angina for 10 years but had managed this well. Despite his loss of work, financial hardship and loss of health he maintained a positive attitude and was thankful for what he described as 'blessings in life'. When visited he was never angry or hopeless and was always kind-hearted.

When asked how he coped with all his problems, particularly his unemployment and financial hardship, he stated that his current unemployment was an opportunity to reflect on his past working life as a milliner and for voluntary work to help others. He saw his 'stay in this world' as being given purpose from God and was thankful that every day over the past 20 years he had been able to find food for himself and his family. He saw God as always there in all stages of his life and believed God took care of him and his family. He was an honest man, respected in his community for his wisdom and positive outlook. He told the nurse that he firmly believed that struggle was the meaning of life, that he continued to do what he could for others as a duty, and that as a Muslim he believed in the grace of Allah. He believed that God tested his believers in different ways but that his own happiness and 'continuing health' showed that God had never left him alone.

Despite his struggle with poverty and ill health for many years, Ibrahim had been sustained by connectedness with his family, his community and his belief in a transcendent God who looked after him. He had a strong sense of purpose and 'becoming'. Life had a clear meaning for him and he felt secure and centred in his being. His positive attitude meant that he did not even perceive himself as suffering.

It possibly reflects the dominant narrative of secular materialism in the affluent West that this is the first narrative we have cited where a positive spiritual attitude, based on religious grounds, has protected not only against material loss and poverty but also against loss of health. We could, of course, cite equally positive narratives of people from other faiths. There are other narratives, too, in which people find their meaning, purpose and even a sense of transcendence through relationships with other people without conscious reference to God. Secular materialism, however, especially if allied to the idolatry of greed, sex or power, may not hold answers to the losses of old age. Interestingly, the otherwise excellent and recommended second edition of *Excellence in Dementia Care* (Downs & Bowers, 2014) deals with many practical aspects of dementia care, including dementia-friendly communities, but makes no mention of spirituality, religion, prayer, churches or even mindfulness in its index.

## Discussion

The six narratives cited in this chapter illustrate in different ways the search for meaning, purpose, connectedness and sometimes transcendence that we associate with the concept of spirituality. Longer narratives written from the points of view of people with dementia (e.g. Rose, 1996; Saunders, 2013) and their carers (e.g. Carling, 2013) are also available. In a culture where the dominant narrative is secular and materialistic, spirituality does not always express itself in or through religion, although our example from the Islamic culture in Pakistan illustrates how a culture in touch with the transcendent can provide rich soil for the development of meaning, purpose and connectedness in a more religious context.

Spiritually competent practice means paying attention to the patient's or carer's narrative 'in the round'. It is assisted by continuity of care so that the patient or carer is enabled to gain from the feeling of personal connection with an empathetic professional or team. Respect for the patient's background culture or religious beliefs is especially relevant when working in a multicultural, multi-faith society, requiring the practitioner to be aware of his or her own world view and spirituality.

Old age is a time of multiple losses, yet most old people cope with remarkable resilience, often based on a lifelong narrative of successfully coping with change and loss. It is undoubtedly enhanced by competent practitioners paying attention to the narrative and to the person, and not just the diagnosis.

## Conclusion

In this chapter we have considered the growing attention being paid to narrative as a tool for learning and good practice, especially in relation to the spiritual challenges of old age. We have considered the relevance of different world views, with their controlling narratives and the individual mindsets based on them. We need to be aware of the (often unexamined) assumptions we make about how the world is and how our assumptions may differ from those of others. Listening to the patient's story enables us to do this and to approach care in a holistic way that does not impose our own cultural assumptions but recognises the importance of helping the patient find meaning and purpose in their unique situation. We have briefly discussed the definition of spirituality, to emphasise how its current use in healthcare embraces secular as well as faith-based approaches, recognising the human need to 'make sense of' and find meaning in life, a need that is often met through narrative approaches. We have highlighted Kang's (2003) description of the six dimensions of psychospiritual integration in discussing the narratives we have given as examples. These have been derived from a variety of practitioners in our multidisciplinary Spirituality Special Interest Group at the University of Huddersfield.

The growing attention now being paid to this area is welcome and we hope the narratives about older adults and how they cope with loss will contribute to an enhanced understanding of how mental health professionals can work together to support them in a spiritually competent way in this essentially spiritual task.

## Acknowledgements

We thank fellow members of the Spirituality Special Interest Group in the School of Human and Health Sciences at the University of Huddersfield who have helped us develop our ideas, especially Gulnar Ali, Ruth Brown, Janice Jones and Melanie Rogers who, along with the authors, have contributed narratives based on their own experiences to this text.

## References

Brooker, D. (2005) Dementia Care Mapping: a review of the research literature. *The Gerontologist*, **45** (special issue 1), 11–18.

Carling, C. (2013) *But Then Something Happened: A Story of Everyday Dementia*. Golden Books.

Cook, C.C.H. (2004) Addiction and spirituality. *Addiction*, **99**, 539–51.

Dew, R. & Koenig, H. (2008) Religion/spirituality and depression in old age. In *Practical Management of Affective Disorders in Older People: A Multi-Professional Approach* (eds S. Curran & J.P. Wattis). Radcliffe Publishers.

Downs, M. & Bowers, B. (eds) (2014) *Excellence in Dementia Care: Research into Practice*, 2nd edn. Open University Press.

Erikson, E.H. (1965) *Childhood and Society*. Penguin Books.

Gordon T., Kelly E. & Mitchell, D. (2011) *Spiritual Care for Healthcare Professionals*. Radcliffe Publishing.

Jewell, A. (1999) *Spirituality and Ageing*. Jessica Kingsley.

Jones, J., Topping, A., Wattis, J., *et al* (2016) A concept analysis of spirituality in occupational therapy practice. *Journal for the Study of Spirituality*, in press.

Kang, C. (2003) A psycho-spiritual integration frame of reference for occupational therapy. Part 1: Conceptual foundations. *Australian Journal of Occupational Therapy*, **50**, 92–103.

Kitwood, T. (1997) *Dementia Reconsidered: The Person Comes First*. Open University Press.

McGrath, A. (2011) *Christian Theology: An Introduction*. Wiley-Blackwell.

Rose, L. (1996) *Show Me the Way to Go Home*. Elder Books.

Saunders, G. (2013) Telling Who I Am before I Forget: My Dementia (excerpt). *The Georgia Review*, Winter. Available at http://garev.uga.edu/winter13/saunders.html (accessed October 2014).

Wallace, D. (2011) Spiritual aspects of dementia. In *Practical Management of Dementia: A Multi-Professional Approach*, 2nd edn (eds S. Curran & J.P. Wattis): pp. 215–28. Radcliffe Publishing.

Wright, N.T. (1992) *The New Testament and the People of God*. SPCK.

CHAPTER 14

# Beginnings and endings

Christopher C. H. Cook, Andrew Powell and Andrew Sims

In Chapter 1, 'Narrative in psychiatry, theology and spirituality', it was suggested that narratives have a beginning and an end. Stories continue, of course, yet at a given point the narrator will have to identify a place to start and a place to stop telling the story. The choice of the beginning and of the ending will significantly frame the narrative and thus influence its impact, meaning and scope. This has been evident throughout the book, with some authors offering narratives that go back to childhood, or narratives that end with a death, but with none that attempts to tell the story of a whole life from birth to death. This is partly due to limitations of space, but it is also because the narratives included have focused primarily on matters of spiritual interest. Of course, if these narrators were to tell the story again after a period of time, they might have more to say, as in the case of a patient who is asked by their doctor 'How have things been since your last appointment?' Each ending of each narration is thus, at least potentially, the beginning of another narrative still to be told.

Importantly, in the present context, every human life must have a beginning and an ending, reflected in its unique narrative, and usually beginning with an account of the family into which a new human life is born. An autobiography generally concludes in the present moment, since the author cannot write, although they may speculate, about what is yet to happen. A biography concludes with a death, and perhaps with a reflection of the enduring impact on the lives of others of a life lived well – or badly.

Each clinical encounter is a privileged opportunity given to the clinician to share in an autobiographical narrative. It usually begins (if told chronologically – which it may well not be) with a history of the family of origin and the personal life history. It must of necessity end in the present moment and it is in the nature of the clinical encounter that both patient and doctor are likely to be speculating about what might happen next. Taking a psychiatric history means listening to the patient's story as well as eliciting the facts; the clinician should also be aware of how the story is presented, what its emphases are, and what it says about the patient's self-identity.

## Spiritual stories

Religious and spiritual traditions have their own narratives. These narratives become interwoven with the lives of those who identify with the tradition, as in the case of the Buddhist seeking enlightenment after the example of Gautama, the Jew who participates in the Passover, or the Christian who is baptised 'into Christ'. Most religious traditions also have some account to give of what happened before our lives began, and what will happen after our lives on this earth have come to an end. They thus have the effect of drawing attention to an earlier beginning, and a more distant end, than might otherwise have received attention.

This wider perspective is not listened to within the clinical context as often or as well as it might be, but it is highly relevant. Thus most mental health chaplains find that one of the most common questions with which they are presented is 'What will happen after I die if I commit suicide?' Yet such things are rarely discussed with a psychiatrist, perhaps for fear of the likely consequences for diagnosis and treatment. The expectation, hope and quest for life after death, whether understood in terms of resurrection, reincarnation or in some other spiritual sense, are widespread human aspirations which significantly influence the way that life is lived in the here and now. They have the effect of turning each possible ending of a human story into a new beginning.

## Narrative and narrator

Other features of narrative identified in Chapter 1 have also recurred throughout the course of the book. A narrative, of necessity, requires a narrator. The primary narrator has almost always been the patient. Yet just the presence of the professional can profoundly influence how the story is told, let alone its being shaped by the questions asked. And when the narrative is retold by the professional, how the narrative has been 'heard' is certain to influence subsequent recollection. Consequently, the professional – be it psychiatrist, chaplain or other health professional – is required to be an attentive listener. This is an art in itself, and essential if the narrator is to tell their story well and to be clearly heard.

If psychiatry has tended to emphasise the taking of a history in a structured way, and if contemporary assessments tend to focus on lists of questions to be asked, then the essays included in this book have tended to affirm stories – as told by patients – that carry a depth of meaning no imposed structure or list can offer. Getting to know people well, whether they are patients or not, is about much more than information obtained by questions. What people include and what they leave out of their stories may sometimes be frustrating to the busy clinician, but it tells us a good deal about what is important to the person. And at their best, these stories are engaging and absorbing. They are also enormously diverse.

Narratives, at least initially, are the prerogative of the narrator. Through narrative, the past, present and future are fashioned into a coherent whole, one in which the past story undergoes selective revision, the present story is chosen and shaped, and the future story is planned. Consequently, the patient as narrator is very much the author of his or her own story. Loss of the sense of control is a problem in almost all forms of mental illness, and narrative helps to gain, and regain, a measure of control – a theme that we encounter throughout this book, notably in Chapter 7, 'Stories of fear: spirituality and anxiety disorders' and Chapter 10, 'My story'.

The chapter authors have used narrative in different ways, yet there are some important common themes, all of which associate narrative with recovery (see Chapter 1, Table 1.1). For example, the very different narratives provided in Chapter 9, 'Narratives of transformation in psychosis' and Chapter 10 chart their own stories of finding identity and meaning in relationship to others and to a vocation in life. Narratives in these and other chapters have also sought to find some kind of understanding of the experience of mental illness. This understanding has usually been facilitated by the mental health professionals concerned, although we have also heard some stories where this has not been the case. Supportive family and friends have featured frequently.

The stories told by patients, families and friends inevitably interweave fact and imagination and consequently have a high index of subjectivity. On the other hand, purely objective assessment is measurement as opposed to story, and while aiming to give a reliable, quantitative profile, it fails to reveal what is most personal in the patient and is of only limited value when deciding on appropriate treatment. Psychiatrists need both subjective and objective accounts from the person they are trying to help. Clinicians should not forget that their own perceptions likewise are subjective – something that holds true even when determining what is intended to be measured objectively.

The teenager with anorexia nervosa and her mother may give completely different accounts of the patient's recent history. This does not have to mean that either is not telling the truth, for their conflicting stories come from different perspectives. The girl may well be trying to describe as accurately as possible how it is for her, while her mother is also trying to give a factual account, but will be hugely influenced by how she experiences her daughter and her illness. The clinician makes 'objective' assessments of weight, physical signs and psychological symptoms, but it may be much harder to understand the internal state of either protagonist. The 'truth' will only be revealed by sympathetically integrating statements and stories from all three persons – mother, daughter and psychiatrist.

The theme of the weaving and interweaving of narratives has been central to this book. The narratives that a person relates of their own experience of mental disorder become woven with the narratives of those close to them, with the narratives of their spiritual and faith tradition, and with the narratives told by mental health professionals. In each case there will be important consequences, for the clinician has the power to facilitate the weaving of narrative in ways that are creative and healing or preside over its un-weaving, with destructive and wounding consequences.

# Beginnings

In Chapter 2, 'Spirituality and transcultural narratives', Simon Dein showed that spirituality, religion and culture are inextricably woven together and that they powerfully influence the way that stories are told. In this interweaving we find not so much the beginning of a narrative – although many religious narratives do include accounts of how things began – but rather the beginnings of particular themes, sub-themes and plots within a larger human story. Thus, in Ayesha's narrative (pp. 17–18), withdrawal, loss of energy and loss of appetite are perceived by her and her family as having their beginning in the spiritual domain, in the activity of the jinn. The same story is perceived by medical staff as having its origins in a depressive illness brought on by childbirth and stress. The resolution of this sub-story within the larger story of Ayesha's life requires a re-weaving of religious and medical narratives in such a way as to produce not only healing but also meaning and reintegration. The task of the physician, and in this case also of the imam, is to facilitate and encourage this weaving and re-weaving of the narrative so as to promote integration and, finally, leave a sense of meaning and purpose about what has happened.

In Chapter 3, 'Psychopathology and the clinical story', Andrew Sims similarly showed that spirituality, religion and psychopathology can become closely, yet not inextricably, interwoven. Here the clinical narrative is an important tool for eliciting the psychopathology that forms a fundamental source of information contributory to making a diagnosis, and thus determining the correct treatment where mental disorder is diagnosed. It is asserted that only skilful un-weaving of the narrative makes it at all possible to talk about separating spirituality and religion on the one hand from psychopathology on the other. In Lucy's story (pp. 36–37), it is possible to discern a strand of narrative that betrays the onset of mental illness and its manifestation in delusional form and content of thought. Intertwined with this is a story of finding a faith that played an important part in helping her to embrace recovery from the illness. The two strands run within a single narrative; as essential aspects of Lucy's autobiography they are inseparable, but as phenomena they can be separated according to form and content and are clearly distinguishable.

In Chapter 4, 'Helping patients tell their story: narratives of body, mind and soul', Andrew Powell showed that in the consulting room, the patient's story becomes the co-creation of therapist and patient working together. The needs of the patient and the aims of the therapist, in ways both obvious and subtle, fashion a narrative from the patient's history and profoundly influence the further story to come. Moving from the objectivity of physical medicine to the subjectivity of mental health, the author describes how, from a profusion of interwoven narratives – societal, biological, pharmaceutical and psychological – the patient can be helped to find his or her authentic self. This is the province of the spiritual narrative, which, having the greater vision, has the power to bestow a new sense of wholeness of being.

Narratives can work for good or ill, as noted in Chapter 1. In Chapter 4, the author concludes by showing how the soul – the spiritual essence of each individual – can be engaged in a therapeutic narrative so that meaning can be conferred on suffering, healing can be encouraged and recovery can begin. This chapter thus introduces a series of chapters within the body of the book in which the transforming power of narrative is explored from different angles.

## Transforming narratives

James Lomax and Ken Pargament show in Chapter 5, 'Gods lost and found: spiritual coping in clinical practice', that narrative can provide both a tool for identifying effective coping resources and a means by which spiritual struggles may be charted and better understood. The management of spiritual struggles proves not so much to be a weaving and re-weaving of strands of a story, but rather the use of narrative to map out new territory and to start telling a new story. In the narrative of Sylvia (pp. 58–59), a diagnosis of depression is found to hide many 'loose ends': a successful professional career that has begun to unravel, a relationship with a father whose expectations Sylvia had only partly lived up to, and suffering encountered in the course of clinical work that raised serious questions about the adequacy for Sylvia of the faith tradition within which she had been raised. In this case, narrative charts new territory – a new story, a new faith community, and a new set of expectations about God, about people and about professional life.

In Chapter 6, 'Stories of joy and sorrow: spirituality and affective disorder', Fred Craigie identifies the important ways in which narrative can help to define and cultivate a sense of purpose in life and to find transcendence. For Craigie purpose means 'living life in faithfulness to deeply important personal values' (p. 70). In particular, people need a reason for living, a reason to engage with recovery. Transcendence '(literally "moving across or rising above some difficulty or obstacle") means being able to "let go" or "make peace" with experiences that are outside of our control' (p. 70). Neither of these factors necessarily need to be understood in spiritual terms but, as Koenig and colleagues (2012: pp. 45–46) have noted, the transcendent is closely connected to concepts of spirituality and religion, and Craigie finds resources within spirituality that are nurturing of both purpose and transcendence.

In Chapter 7, 'Stories of fear: spirituality and anxiety disorders', Chris Williams identifies narrative as the milieu within which cognitive–behavioural therapy can take place. The process of transformation that is described here is based on changing the interpretation of that which is perceived as threat, and (like Lomax and Pargament) on building coping skills. Within this process of transformation, spirituality and religion may, or may not, play an important part according to the needs of the person being treated. Narrative here is less about charting new territory, less about finding purpose and transcendent connection, and more about providing a framework within which spiritual concerns and resources can be located alongside other significant resources in support of a process of change.

In Chapter 8, 'Stories of transgression: narrative therapy with offenders', Gwen Adshead writes of seeking to 'transform narratives of cruelty and madness into narratives of regret and hope'. Narrative here is both a therapeutic tool – the means of transformation – and the focus of transformation, which she sees as being at the heart of the recovery process. Narratives can be coherent, communicating 'a message with meaning in a fresh, authentic and reflective way', or incoherent, being not so much incomprehensible and incomplete as confusing. Narrative therapies address these deficits so as to facilitate the discovery of a new way of being, one that both owns the reality of the past and offers hope for the future. Like Powell, Adshead finds that this process has much in common with spirituality:

> 'What I perceive the narrative and the spiritual to have in common is an inquiring stance that assumes that humans want to make meaning of their actions and lives, if they can; and I assume that stance is also consistent with most forms of psychotherapeutic enquiry' (p. 94).

In Chapter 9, 'Narratives of transformation in psychosis', Isabel Clarke presents the radical argument that narratives of psychosis are narratives of transformation. In support of this, three contributors share their own experience of mental illness. Using the concept of 'high schizotypy' (not to be confused with schizotypal personality disorder), Clarke seeks to normalise 'openness to the unusual and the anomalous that lie beyond consensual reality'. She writes:

> 'The concern of this chapter has been with a way of experiencing open to all human beings but more often accessed by high schizotypes. This has been the territory of saints and mystics; they too encountered terror as well as ecstasy, their experiences were frequently preceded by illness or transition, and their day-to-day functioning was often supported by a community when compromised' (pp. 115–116).

Many psychiatrists will be sceptical of the views expressed in this chapter, and even those sympathetic to this approach may nevertheless argue with such a broad assertion. Notably, the narratives provided here are of relatively mild and atypical accounts of psychosis. Theologians, too, may be concerned about equating the experiences of saints and mystics with those of psychosis (Cook, 2012). Nonetheless, the narratives of Katie, Satyin and Hilary are striking testimony to their tenacity and authenticity in a spiritual quest for deeper meaning and relationship.

The accounts provided in Chapter 9 contrast with Jo Barber's personal narrative in Chapter 10. Barber's story is also one of finding meaning and purpose in psychosis, but only through struggle and with the help of others, including chaplaincy and mental health professionals. It is a transformation through acknowledging the need to disentangle the spiritual from the psychopathological rather than conflating them. As a result of this disentangling (cf. Chapter 3), a place of integration of spiritual and religious well-being is eventually found. Within the story may be found the importance of searching for meaning (cf. Chapter 4), new beginnings (cf. Chapter 5), experiences of transcendence (cf. Chapter 6) and the healing power of narrative itself (cf. Chapter 8). Barber provides a moving account both of the depths of despair with which mental illness can be associated and of the courage and perseverance with which recovery may be pursued. Within the vicissitudes of this narrative, spirituality plays a key part in the recovery that is eventually achieved.

In Chapter 11, 'God's story revealed in the human story', similarly, there is an account of transformation through suffering. Here, Beaumont Stevenson shows how narrative grounded in the seemingly small events of everyday life has the capacity to acquire a deeper significance and to embrace a greater reality. He draws on his wide experience of mental health chaplaincy to describe how patients, in ways often unforeseen and unexpected, and in the midst of their suffering, are given to gestures of kindness and compassion. Stevenson's skill is to respond to those moments as they arise with symbol and metaphor, conjuring the bigger picture and so bringing the individual who suffers in isolation into relation with others. Becoming part of humanity once again, people discover they belong to more than themselves and together, on this larger stage, it becomes possible to move beyond personal pain and to rediscover hope, meaning and purpose. Stevenson intimates that this transformation from the meaningless to the meaningful, from despair to hope, and from isolation to connection is the divine story manifest in humanity, where the awakening of love is the key to the restoration and healing of the human spirit.

In Chapters 10 and 11, and elsewhere in this book, the spirituality of transformation is mediated through a Christian narrative. In Chapter 12, 'Meaning without believing: attachment theory, mentalisation and the spiritual dimension of analytical psychotherapy', Jeremy Holmes, a 'non-believer', argues that spirituality is implicitly woven into the practice of dynamic psychotherapy. He highlights both the importance of emotions that uplift and the need to face pain and suffering – as avowed by religion and spirituality. He points to the importance of current research into mentalising, which he refers to as 'the capacity to stand back from oneself and one's thoughts and to question them' (p. 150). This capacity to reflect upon experiences of both joy and sorrow facilitates a spiritual approach to life, recognising its mystery (including the transcendent) and accepting with humility that there is much we cannot know. Turning to attachment theory (while leaving aside the question of whether God actually exists), Holmes asks how secure attachment might relate to the Buddhist practice of non-attachment. His answer is that at best the one can enable the other. Similarly, while mindfulness could be used to defend against working with the meaning of depressive thoughts (i.e. anti-mentalising), when used well, it encourages 'a decentred, negativity-defusing perspective' (p. 152). Holmes concludes that psychotherapy 'is no more and no less than an intensely practical and loving pathway to spiritual aliveness' (p. 158).

## Endings

In Chapter 13, 'Stories of living with loss: spirituality and ageing', John Wattis and Steven Curran highlight the particular challenges of later life and the many losses that advancing age brings. Here, the emphasis moves from transformation to endings. Losses through bereavement, divorce, retirement, illness, failing strength or mental faculties, or having to face the prospect of a foreshortened life are all endings of different kinds. Later life can bring new opportunities and new relationships, but the capacity to enter into these fully and happily requires a person to negotiate successfully the concomitant endings. Decline, both physical and mental, including the impact of dementia, brings an irreversibility that the relentless passage of time only serves to accentuate. How this is understood or experienced has profound spiritual implications, whether interpreted through traditional religious or atheistic or agnostic narratives, each of which offers a different framework of meaning. The narratives given here unfold in diverse ways, not all obviously spiritual, let alone religious; they include hobbies such as gardening and playing the piano, relationships with family and community (including faith community), living in the present moment, and keeping a positive mental attitude. The authors show how secular spirituality can provide solace and how holistic care based on attending to a person's specific needs can enable someone in the twilight of life to find and express their spirituality, described here within a framework of becoming, meaning, being, centredness, connectedness and transcendence.

## Conclusions

As we reach the end of this book, what conclusions might we draw about spirituality, narrative and the clinical practice of psychiatry?

First, narrative seems to provide a conducive medium for the formation, transformation, expression and communication of spiritual and religious concerns. This may be for a variety of reasons. One aspect of spirituality concerns the interpretation of narrative so that a greater meaning emerges from the lesser. A telling of the narrative is thus an essential first step in the process, but importantly, it also allows the listener to form their own conclusions – to make their own interpretations and find their own meaning as they see fit. It invites discussion, which thus fosters communication about things that are important, and through this process, the spiritual narrative enables the narrator to clarify and give shape to fundamental concerns such as transcendence, relationship, meaning and purpose.

Second, narratives frequently employ metaphors, symbols, images and motifs. These, in turn, point to other concerns not easily conveyed in spoken or written language (being more or less ineffable). There may be allusions to religious narratives, to myths or to other archetypal themes that interweave with the narrative itself, enriching it, adding layers of meaning and enhancing its significance. This weaving and interweaving conveys a sense of the narrative as bound up within the wider human story, making each individual life part of something much bigger and altogether more important.

Third, narratives convey much of the most important information that is essential to the clinical task – the history and psychopathology on which diagnosis and treatment are based. Clinicians endeavour to record this information in other ways, including structured interviews, questionnaires, and computerised assessments, all of which attempt to provide systematic and comprehensive logging of information while guarding against blame for failure to ask key questions. Yet these approaches do not in themselves offer a compassionate, human or patient-centred account of what has been going on and, furthermore, they are liable to their own inaccuracies. Largely focused on the concerns of the clinician, they serve to arrive at a diagnosis rather than helping to understand another human being. Narrative, in contrast, far surpasses quantitative measurement at elucidating many, perhaps most, of the complex facts with which human lives are concerned.

Fourth, narrative clearly has a special place in all 'talking therapies'. Since 2010, the UK National Health Service has been resourcing the Improving Access to Psychological Therapies (IAPT) programme in response to a strong evidence base as well as the expressed wish of patients to be helped in this way. Narrative is here to stay, for it is at the heart of the psychotherapeutic process, and of the recovery movement in mental healthcare. People find it helpful to tell their stories. They feel better for doing so, which in turn makes it easier to cope with adversity.

How is this relevant to spirituality? This volume has been concerned to show that spirituality, understood broadly, is concerned with finding meaning and purpose and, more than that, inspiring a person to accomplish what they have in them to be. For all these reasons, narrative offers much that can enrich psychiatric best practice. Why then is narrative not found more commonly at the heart of the clinical process? Fears of litigation, of missing something important that should have been specifically asked about, or of leaving the patient (as narrator) with too much power over the assessment process may all play their part. Lack of understanding of the value and importance of narrative in clinical training – at undergraduate and postgraduate level – is probably also significant; regrettably, the skills of storytelling and listening to stories are rarely taught.

A further crucial factor that militates against narrative is the sheer pressure on mental health services today. The narrating of stories, and listening to them well, takes time – and time is in short supply in an increasingly pressurised and closely governed health service. If this were not enough, the psychiatrist who is concerned to offer person-centred care has to cope with a culture in which mental health science is more interested in investigating the objective (the 'I-it' of which Martin Buber (1937) writes) than in recognising the value of the inter-subjective (the 'I-Thou'). The danger is too much 'doing to' and too little 'being with'. This mirrors a wider societal trend, in which people are losing touch with the inner world, both their own and that of others. The effect is an impoverishment of spirit, a dullness of the senses, an inability to savour life – something the psychiatrist sees day after day.

What is to be done? We have set out to show, through a range of clinical perspectives, that paying close attention to the patient's story is not a luxury but the foundation of good psychiatric practice. Patients' spiritual or religious beliefs, so often neglected by psychiatrists, are to be found embedded in their stories and once discerned can be readily elicited. It has been the aim of this book to show how awareness of the spiritual narrative can significantly improve how psychiatrists help their patients, something we recognise that has implications both for the training and the continuing professional development of the profession.

To conclude with a narrative from the 13th century, what might the esteemed friar St Francis of Assisi advise, were he alive today? While suffering greatly from physical illness, St Francis wrote the *Canticle of the Creatures*. He indicated that he wished to 'compose a new hymn about the Lord's creatures, of which we make daily use, without which we cannot live, and with which the human race greatly offends its Creator' (Armstrong *et al*, 1999: p. 113). The *Canticle* considers simple but important things that we often take for granted – things that are beautiful, useful and significant but which we have stopped noticing because they are always there. Each in turn is personified by St Francis so as to remind us of the virtues that it conveys, and which we would do well to imitate. Thus, Brother Sun is praised for giving us light, likewise Sister Mother Earth who 'sustains and governs' us, and not least Sister Water, 'who is very useful and humble and precious and chaste'.

Narrative, like Sister Water, is useful, humble, precious and yet simple, a tool of human communication that in healthcare is all too frequently overlooked. The clinician who understands its value and puts it to use will find that narrative transforms the mechanical task of collecting information into meaningful, heartfelt dialogue; one that has the power to effect healing and relieve suffering.

# References

Armstrong, R.J., Hellmann, J.A.W., & Short, W.J. (1999) *Francis of Assisi – The saint.* I. Early Documents. New City Press.

Buber, M. (1937) *I and Thou.* T&T Clark.

Cook, C.C.H. (2012) Psychiatry in scripture: sacred texts and psychopathology. *The Psychiatrist,* **36**, 225–9.

Koenig, H.G., King, D.E. & Carson, V.B. (2012) *Handbook of Religion and Health,* 2nd edn. Oxford University Press.

# Index

## Compiled by Linda English

abstractions 7, 11
addiction: theological model 35–36
aetiology 39, 40–41
affective disorder: and spirituality 67–81, 177
  acceptance/willingness 76
  'all I have to do' exercise 74–75
  compassionate presence 69–70
  conversational approaches to purpose 72–74
  exercises in defining purpose 74–75
  forgiveness 69, 78
  'going away celebration' exercise 74
  gratitude/gratefulness 77–78
  healing intention 69–70
  language 73, 74
  letting go 76
  mindfulness/being present 76–77
  moving forward with purpose 75
  narrative in spiritual care 69–70
  non-attachment 77
  'patient wisdom' and 'clinician wisdom' 75
  purpose 70–75
  self-reflective practices 79
  serenity 77
  'someone who loves you' exercise 74
  spirituality 68–69
  staying connected 79
  'three adjectives' exercise 74
  transcendence 70–75
  vital and sacred 70, 74
  'you at your best' exercise 74–75
  see also depression
affirmations 79
African–Caribbeans in UK: charismatic Christianity 21–22
ageing: and spirituality 160–172, 180
  loss 160, 162–170
  narrative in context 160–161
  narratives 163–170

  psychiatric history 160
  resilience 162
  world views 160–161
alcohol addiction 10, 35–36
Alcoholics Anonymous 10, 95, 133
altruism 148, 157
analytical psychotherapy: spiritual dimension 145–159, 179–180
anxiety disorders: and spirituality 82–93, 177–178
  anxiety balance 83
  CBT and faith aspects 82–92
  five areas assessment 90, 91
  narrative approach 82–83
  narratives 84–92
Aristotle: *Metaphysics* 48
arousal management 117
attachment 58, 60, 94
  disorganised 102, 148, 156
  God 54, 148–149, 151, 155
  non-attachment 77, 155–156, 180
  psychotherapy 145–146, 148–149, 151, 152, 155, 156–157, 158, 180
  spirituality 148–149
auditory hallucinations 32, 44
authentic narrative 43
autobiographical narrative 8, 9, 173

Bangladeshi narratives 17–19
bereavement 50, 71, 100, 149, 165
Bible 31, 92, 139
bipolar disorder 31, 37, 40–41, 57, 108
body/mind/soul narratives 39–52, 176–177
both/and logic 115, 116, 118
Buddhism 48, 112, 150, 155, 174
Bunyan: *Pilgrim's Progress* 6

CBT *see* cognitive–behavioural therapy
chaos narrative 3

# INDEX

charismatic Christianity: UK African–
  Caribbeans 21–22
Christianity 26, 30, 174, 179
  Bible 31, 92, 139
  CBT and anxiety disorders 87–92
  charismatic among UK African–
    Caribbeans 21–22
  confession/repentance/redemption 104
  crucifix 140
  desert experience 132–133
  gratitude 77
  Jesus 6, 135, 136, 138, 140, 153, 155
  mystics 33, 105
  sacrifice 155
  service user's spiritual narrative 121–130
  speaking in tongues 44
  spirituality and psychotherapy 154
  *see also* God
clinical story: and psychopathology 25–38, 176
co-creation of narrative: by therapist and patient 43
cognitions: religious 35
cognitive architecture model 115
cognitive–behavioural therapy (CBT)
  anxiety disorders 82–93, 177–178
  psychosis 116
communities 79
concrete thinking 29–30, 44, 141
confession: offenders 104–105
consciousness 47–48
content: and form 26, 27, 32–33, 176
contractions 7
conversational maxims 97–98, 99
coping
  anxiety balance 83
  old age 163–170
  spiritual *see* spiritual coping
countertransference 62
creation narrative 7
creedal statements 35
culture 14
  avoid cultural stereotyping 16
  controlling narratives 161
  cross-cultural narratives of mental illness 14–15
  multi-cultural society 161, 170
  religion and 16
  spirituality and transcultural narratives 14–24
  world views 160–161

death: life after 174
delusions 26, 28, 29, 32, 34, 110, 138–139, 176

dementia 167–169, 170
Dementia Care Mapping 168
demonic possession 21, 123
depression 3, 25, 46, 92, 96
  major 41
  mindfulness-based cognitive therapy 152
  old age 163–164, 166
  spirituality and affective disorder 67–81, 177
  spiritual struggles 58–59
  transcultural narratives 15, 18, 20, 21, 176
descriptive phenomenology 25–27, 28
desert experience 132–133, 134
diagnosis 5
  descriptive psychopathology 29
  diagnostic narrative 40
  pre-eminence of medical diagnosis 39–40
  of psychosis 118
*Diagnostic and Statistical Manual of Mental Disorders* (DSM) 28, 41
dissociative state 33–34
dreaming 146–147

eating disorders 137–138, 175
ego 43, 48
  ego-less states 146–147
empathy 25–26
equivalence mode: non-mentalising 150, 152
Excellence in Dementia Care 170
exercise 79
exorcism 123, 124

faith
  CBT and anxiety support 83–92
  phenomenology of 34–36
family therapy 142
father idealization 137–138
fluoxetine (Prozac) 41
forgiveness 50–51, 69, 78
form: and content 26, 27, 32–33, 176
Freud, S. 42, 54, 146, 157

generativity 62
God 20, 31, 48, 50, 61, 86–87, 149
  archetypal Imago Dei 48, 49
  attachment 54, 148–149, 151, 155
  father and 58, 59
  God's narrative 11
  Islamic 48, 169
  love of 152
  Moses and 136–137
  revealed in human story 132–144
  service user's spiritual narrative 121–130
  spiritual struggles 57

**186**

## INDEX

gratitude journals 77–78
group therapy 44, 101, 133
guest narrator 137

hallucinations 8, 32, 44, 45, 115
*Handbook of Spiritual Care in Mental Illness* 128
Hasidic Judaism 19–21
healing 2
heart 50–51
　distress 14–15
　sinking 15
heroes 95, 96, 112
Hinduism 48
Hoffman, Melchior 33
Holocaust survivors 103, 149
home-study programme: spirituality 68
homicide 44, 94, 95, 99, 100, 101–102, 103–104

I-it 139, 182
illness 12
　chronic/terminal 3, 16–17, 39–40
　differs from disease 133
　journey 3
　narratives 2–4, 21
　old age 163, 169–170
　self and 133–134
impermanence 150–151, 155
Improving Access to Psychological Therapies (IAPT) programme 181
*International Classification of Diseases* (ICD) 28, 41, 44
Islam 16, 17–18, 48, 77, 84–86, 132, 169
I-Thou 139, 147, 182

Jaspers, Karl 25–26, 32
Jesus 6, 135, 136, 138, 140, 153, 155
jinn possession 17–18, 123, 176
journals 77–78, 79
Judaism 77, 149, 174
　Bible 31
　CBT and anxiety disorders 86–87
　desert experience 132–133
　Hasidic 19–21
　narratives 19–21
Julian of Norwich 33, 46

Kempe, Margery 8–9

late paraphrenia 31
life history book 168–169
'living human documents' 6, 8
locus of control
　external 27
　internal 27, 30

mass suicide 44
meaning 2, 6, 8, 10, 62, 94
　dimension of spirituality 161
　old age 161, 165, 171
　phenomenology 26
　transcultural narratives 17
　without believing 145–159
medicine
　medical model 27
　narrative in 1–5, 26
　psychiatry and 40–41
mental disorders: burden of disease/disability 41
Mental Health Act 11, 22, 45
mental health chaplains 34, 113, 118, 127, 128, 134–135, 138, 174
mentalising 157–158, 179
　mystery and 149–152
　three non-mentalising modes 150–151, 152
metaphors 135, 136, 141, 181
metaphysical *v.* physicalist view 47–48
mindfulness 69, 76–77, 79, 116, 117, 152, 180
mindfulness-based cognitive therapy (MBCT) 152
motivational interviewing 118
motivations: religious and spiritual 55
music 122, 124, 129
mysticism 8, 10, 33, 105, 115–116, 117, 146, 150, 178

nafs ('lower self') 16
narrative
　beginnings and endings 173–183
　coherence of 97–99
　harmful narratives 2, 4, 44
　in medicine 1–5, 26
　narrative-based *v.* evidence-based medicine 26
　narrator and 1, 174–176
　in psychiatry 1–5
　in spirituality 5–9
　in theology 5–9
　*see also* spiritual narrative; story/stories
narrative therapy: with offenders *see* offenders
narrator 1, 174–176
Nebuchadnezzar 31
negative affect 137–138, 147, 148, 152, 154, 157
neurotic disorders 27
Newtonian mechanics 47

'O' 146
obsessional disorder 21, 86–87

**187**

# INDEX

offenders: narrative therapy 94–107, 178
  anxiety 102, 103
  childhood adversity 102
  coherence of narrative 97–99
  confession, repentance and redemption 104–105
  conversational maxims 97–98, 99
  group work 101
  language 94–95, 96–97, 103
  narratives of offending 96–97
  narratives and recovery 95–96, 99–101
  problems with narrative approaches 102–104
  sense of agency 97
  spirituality 104–105
  transformation and redemption 101–102
old age *see* ageing: and spiritualty
Omar Khayyám 43
organic diseases 31, 40
organisational culture 161
overvalued idea 33

panic attacks 42
parent/child dynamic 43
passivity experience 25, 27, 32
pathological interpretation: spirituality and religion 11
Pentecostalism 21
pharmaceutical narrative: of mental disorders 41
phenomenology
  descriptive 25–27, 28
  of faith 34–6
  with spirituality 36–7
  of therapeutic spirituality 145–148
poverty 169–170
power: abuse of 42
prayer 68, 77, 86, 135
Present State Examination 27, 28
pretend mode: non-mentalising 150–151, 152
psychiatric history 160, 173
psychiatrists 5–6, 17, 28, 32, 35, 39, 47, 49, 175
psychiatry 40–42
  narrative in medicine and 1–5
  spiritual narratives in 9–11
psychoanalysis 42–43, 146, 147, 154, 157
psychopathology 8, 45
  can spiritual/religious experiences be distinguished from 27–30
  clinical story and 25–38, 176
  descriptive 40–41
  dynamic 42–43

form and content 26, 27, 32–33
phenomenology of faith 34–36
phenomenology with spirituality 36–7
religious 31–4
'religious patients' 31–4
psychosis 25, 36–37, 55, 141
  acute and transient 45–46
  Kraepelin's classification 40
  narratives of transformation in 108–120, 178–179
  offenders 99, 102
  problem-solving model 114
  psychotic narrative 44
  spiritual/religious experience and 27–30, 31, 45–46
psychotherapy 42–43, 49, 60, 62–63, 68, 94, 181
  ego-less states 146–147
  enhanced spirituality as outcome 153–154
  narrative therapy with offenders 94–107
  positive emotions 147–148
  spiritual dimension of analytical 145–159, 179–180
  as spirituality 152–153
  spirituality as alternative to 151–152
  spirituality beyond 154–155
  transcendent experiences 145–146
puerperal psychosis 8

quantum field theory 47–48
quest narrative 3, 9
Qur'anic recitations 17, 18

recovery 9–10, 47
  narrative 3–4, 10, 45, 95–96, 175
  offenders 95–96, 99–101
redemption 7
  offenders 95, 96, 101–102, 104–105
refugees 17
religion 5–9
  beliefs 30, 34–36
  cross-cultural use of term problematic 16
  culture and 16
  Freud on 54
  mystery 149
  psychiatric symptoms *v.* religious experience 27–30, 126
  recovery and 9–10
  'religiosity gap' 5
  service user's spiritual narrative 121–130
  ubiquity in human societies 148
  *see also* below and individual religions
religious
  cognitions 35
  conversion 153

delusions 29, 34, 138–139
experience 22, 27–30, 34
narrative 3, 10
observance 20–21
psychopathology 31–34
'religious patients' 31–34
repentance: offenders 104–105
restitution narrative 3, 11
resurrection narrative 7
retreats: spiritual 68, 79
Royal College of Psychiatrists 5–6, 47, 113
*ruh* (soul) 16

St Augustine: *Confessions* 6
St Francis of Assisi: *Canticle of the Creatures* 182
St John of the Cross 46
 *Dark Night* 10
St Louis of Gonzaga 33
Saul 45
schizophrenia 40–41, 45–46, 108
 African–Caribbeans in UK 22
 concrete thinking 29–30, 44
 first rank symptoms 32
 recovery 95
 religious psychopathology 34
 spiritual coping 54–55, 57
 in traditional societies 115
schizotypy: high schizotypes 114, 115–116, 178
science narrative: and spirituality narrative 47–48
secularism 149, 161, 169–170
self-identity 2, 11
serenity prayer 77
service user's narrative 121–131, 179
sexual abuse 56, 69
shamanic role 141–142
sin 20, 21
societal narrative 41
somatization 15, 18
soul 16, 47, 67
 narrative 39, 48–51, 176–177
South Asians in UK 18
speaking in tongues ('Toronto blessing') 44
spiritual
 care 68–70, 128
 emergence 110
 emergency 112
 experience *v.* psychiatric symptoms 27–30, 45–46
 history 47
spiritual coping 53–66, 177
 clinical narratives 57–62
 functions 54–55

many methods of 55
prevalence 53–54
spiritual struggles 55–57, 58, 62–63, 177
theory and research 53–57
Spiritual Crisis Network 108, 110
spirituality 12
 affective disorder and 67–81, 177
 analytical psychotherapy and 145–159
 anxiety disorders and 82–93, 177–178
 attachment theory and 148–149
 definition 5, 70, 94, 161–162
 in Islam 16
 offenders and 104–105
 phenomenology with 36–37
 six dimensions of 161–162, 163
 transcultural narratives and 14–24
 without religion 36, 46, 48
spiritual narrative 3, 5–9, 45–48, 49, 69–70
 dreams 147
 healing 136–140
 living in eternal now 136–137
 in mental health community 134–135
 metaphor 136
 in psychiatry 9–11
 reframing delusional 138–139
 science narrative and 47–48
 service user's story 121–131
 suffering 140
 symbol 136
 transformation of I-it into I-Thou 139
 'writing' new story 137–138
story/stories
 cultural locus 14
 of fear 82–93
 God's 132–144
 living with loss 160–172
 mundane 6, 7
 psychopathology and clinical story 25–38
 quest 95
 sacred 6–7
 service user's 121–131
 spiritual 174
 storytelling 1, 78, 140
 of transgression 94–107
stressors 53–54, 55
stroke 163
subjectivity/objectivity 175
sublimation 147
suffering 41–42, 140, 142, 154, 155, 157–158
suicide 50, 74, 109
 life after death 174
 mass 44
 offenders 99, 100, 101
 service user's narrative 125, 126
symbols 136, 141, 181

**189**

# INDEX

teleological thinking: non-mentalising mode 150, 152
theology
  narrative in 5–9
  theological model of addiction 35–36
  theological reflection 8, 11
Torah 19, 20, 21
traditional healers 17, 18
training needed 63–64
trance states 44
transcendence 6, 145–146, 162, 167, 177
transcultural narratives: and spirituality 14–24, 176
  Bangladeshi narratives 17–19
  charismatic Christianity among UK African–Caribbeans 21–22
  cross-cultural narratives of mental illness 14–15

Jewish narratives 19–21
narratives in clinical practice 16–17
spiritual and religious narratives 15–16
transforming narratives 177–180
  in psychosis 108–120, 178

unconscious 42, 151, 156, 157

volition 35–36

well-being
  dementia 169
  spiritual and religious 121–123, 124, 127, 128–129
'What is Real and What is Not' group 116
witchcraft 17, 18